BIOMEDICAL ETHICS

Opposing Viewpoints®

Roman Espejo, *Book Editor*

Daniel Leone, *President*
Bonnie Szumski, *Publisher*
Scott Barbour, *Managing Editor*

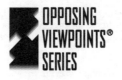

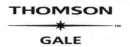

San Diego • Detroit • New York • San Francisco • Cleveland
New Haven, Conn. • Waterville, Maine • London • Munich

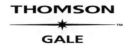

LIBRARY OF CONGRESS CATALOGING-IN-PUBLICATION DATA
Biomedical ethics / Roman Espejo, book editor.
p. cm. — (Opposing viewpoints)
Includes bibliographical references and index.
ISBN 0-7377-1219-8 (pbk. : alk. paper) — ISBN 0-7377-1220-1 (lib. : alk. paper)
1. Medical ethics. 2. Bioethics—Philosophy. 3. Bioethics. I. Espejo, Roman,
1977– II. Opposing viewpoints series (Unnumbered)
R725.5 .B55 2003
174'.2—dc21   2002023258

"Congress shall make no law...abridging the freedom of speech, or of the press."

First Amendment to the U.S. Constitution

The basic foundation of our democracy is the First Amendment guarantee of freedom of expression. The Opposing Viewpoints Series is dedicated to the concept of this basic freedom and the idea that it is more important to practice it than to enshrine it.

Contents

Why Consider Opposing Viewpoints?

"The only way in which a human being can make some approach to knowing the whole of a subject is by hearing what can be said about it by persons of every variety of opinion and studying all modes in which it can be looked at by every character of mind. No wise man ever acquired his wisdom in any mode but this."

John Stuart Mill

In our media-intensive culture it is not difficult to find differing opinions. Thousands of newspapers and magazines and dozens of radio and television talk shows resound with differing points of view. The difficulty lies in deciding which opinion to agree with and which "experts" seem the most credible. The more inundated we become with differing opinions and claims, the more essential it is to hone critical reading and thinking skills to evaluate these ideas. Opposing Viewpoints books address this problem directly by presenting stimulating debates that can be used to enhance and teach these skills. The varied opinions contained in each book examine many different aspects of a single issue. While examining these conveniently edited opposing views, readers can develop critical thinking skills such as the ability to compare and contrast authors' credibility, facts, argumentation styles, use of persuasive techniques, and other stylistic tools. In short, the Opposing Viewpoints Series is an ideal way to attain the higher-level thinking and reading skills so essential in a culture of diverse and contradictory opinions.

In addition to providing a tool for critical thinking, Opposing Viewpoints books challenge readers to question their own strongly held opinions and assumptions. Most people form their opinions on the basis of upbringing, peer pressure, and personal, cultural, or professional bias. By reading carefully balanced opposing views, readers must directly confront new ideas as well as the opinions of those with whom they disagree. This is not to simplistically argue that everyone who reads opposing views will—or should—change his or her opinion. Instead, the series enhances readers' understanding of their own views by encouraging confrontation with opposing ideas. Careful examination of others' views can lead to the readers' understanding of the logical inconsistencies in their own opinions, perspective on why they hold an opinion, and the consideration of the possibility that their opinion requires further evaluation.

Evaluating Other Opinions

To ensure that this type of examination occurs, Opposing Viewpoints books present all types of opinions. Prominent spokespeople on different sides of each issue as well as well-known professionals from many disciplines challenge the reader. An additional goal of the series is to provide a forum for other, less known, or even unpopular viewpoints. The opinion of an ordinary person who has had to make the decision to cut off life support from a terminally ill relative, for example, may be just as valuable and provide just as much insight as a medical ethicist's professional opinion. The editors have two additional purposes in including these less known views. One, the editors encourage readers to respect others' opinions—even when not enhanced by professional credibility. It is only by reading or listening to and objectively evaluating others' ideas that one can determine whether they are worthy of consideration. Two, the inclusion of such viewpoints encourages the important critical thinking skill of objectively evaluating an author's credentials and bias. This evaluation will illuminate an author's reasons for taking a particular stance on an issue and will aid in readers' evaluation of the author's ideas.

It is our hope that these books will give readers a deeper understanding of the issues debated and an appreciation of the complexity of even seemingly simple issues when good and honest people disagree. This awareness is particularly important in a democratic society such as ours in which people enter into public debate to determine the common good. Those with whom one disagrees should not be regarded as enemies but rather as people whose views deserve careful examination and may shed light on one's own.

Thomas Jefferson once said that "difference of opinion leads to inquiry, and inquiry to truth." Jefferson, a broadly educated man, argued that "if a nation expects to be ignorant and free . . . it expects what never was and never will be." As individuals and as a nation, it is imperative that we consider the opinions of others and examine them with skill and discernment. The Opposing Viewpoints Series is intended to help readers achieve this goal.

David L. Bender and Bruno Leone,
Founders

Greenhaven Press anthologies primarily consist of previously published material taken from a variety of sources, including periodicals, books, scholarly journals, newspapers, government documents, and position papers from private and public organizations. These original sources are often edited for length and to ensure their accessibility for a young adult audience. The anthology editors also change the original titles of these works in order to clearly present the main thesis of each viewpoint and to explicitly indicate the opinion presented in the viewpoint. These alterations are made in consideration of both the reading and comprehension levels of a young adult audience. Every effort is made to ensure that Greenhaven Press accurately reflects the original intent of the authors included in this anthology.

Introduction

"If you are criticizing genetic engineering then you are cutting off the only humane way for mankind out of regress."

— *Edward Kinitz,* Why Genetic Engineering
Is Advantageous for Humankind, *2000*

"Humans have long since possessed the tools for crafting a better world. Where love, compassion, altruism and justice have failed, genetic manipulation will not succeed."

— *Gina Maranto,* Quest for Perfection:
The Drive to Breed Better Humans, *1996*

Leilani Muir was one of nearly 2,900 people involuntarily sterilized between 1928 and 1972 in Alberta, Canada. When Muir reached adolescence, her fallopian tubes were removed without her knowledge or consent. She was subjected to the procedure because a law permitted the Alberta government to sterilize mentally deficient individuals to prevent the birth of similarly afflicted children. As a child, Muir had scored 67 on an IQ test, an indication of subnormal human intelligence. (However, later IQ tests concluded that she possessed normal human intelligence.) In 1995, Muir finally came forward and became the first victim of the long-defunct policy to sue the Alberta government for wrongful sterilization. She won her lawsuit—government lawyers agreed that Muir was entitled to damages because she was unable to reverse her sterility. However, they asserted that her victory did not indicate that the government was liable for other sterilization cases. Nonetheless, dozens of victims of the sterilization law sought damages from the Alberta government thereafter.

Using sterilization in order to reduce the births of children with undesirable traits is among the numerous ways of achieving the goal of eugenics. Meaning "good in birth" in Greek (*eu*: good, *genos*: birth), eugenics refers to the practice of attempting to improve the human race through selective breeding. The origins of modern eugenics can be traced to the late nineteenth century. Sir Francis Galton, a cousin of evolutionary theorist Charles Darwin, coined the term in 1883. While studying a population sample of British subjects, Galton noted that exceptionally intelligent and talented individuals were disproportionately related to each other. Consequently, he concluded that such characteristics were hereditary and identified two principal means of genetically improving the human race—through "positive" and "negative" eugenics. In positive eugenics, individuals with "good" genetic stock, or desirable mental and physical traits, are encouraged to marry each other and reproduce. In negative eugenics, individuals with "bad" genetic stock, or undesirable traits, are discouraged from reproducing. Historically, the objectives of positive and negative eugenics have been pursued primarily through segregation and sterilization.

Although it is infamously associated with Nazi Germany's attempt to exterminate the Jewish race, eugenics has shaped the laws and policies in different nations, both in the past and the present. For example, in the late–nineteenth century United States, the wave of immigrants from eastern and southern Europe was widely perceived as a threat to American society. They were thought to carry bad genetic stock because disparate numbers of eastern and southern European immigrants committed crimes and populated poverty-stricken areas. As a result, twenty-four of America's states enacted eugenics-based sterilization laws, targeting ethnic minorities, the poor, and the "feeble-minded" in order to reduce crime and poverty. In fact, by 1933, California had sterilized more people for eugenic purposes than all other states combined. Although these American laws disappeared by the mid–twentieth century, eugenics-based policies can be found in different parts of the world. For instance, in 1994, the Singapore government introduced eugenics-based family planning, offering the poor and uneducated financial incentives to undergo sterilization after having one or two children to reduce their burden on society.

Advances in genetic engineering have transformed the eugenics debate by raising the possibility of eugenics via genetic manipulation. Two types of cells in mammals—somatic cells and germline cells—carry genetic material and can be modified during the embryonic stage to change the characteristics of an organism. However, there is a fundamental difference between engineering somatic cells and germline cells. If an embryo's somatic cells, or nonreproductive cells such as skin or muscle cells, are modified, only the organism will be changed. The changes to its genes will not be passed on to its offspring. But if an embryo's germline cells, or reproductive cells, are modified, the organism's changes are inheritable—subsequent generations will inherit the genetic modification. Therefore, germline genetic engineering may enable human beings to control their own genetic makeup and usher a new age of eugenics.

Supporters of eugenics take into account the brutal acts of inhumanity that have been committed for the sake of ethnic cleansing and "improving" the human race. However, many of them argue that a clear distinction lies between using genetics technology to reach social, racial, and political ends and allowing a willing, informed person to use genetic technology for themselves and their children. For example, bioethicists Arthur L. Caplan, Glenn McGee, and David Magnus support the use of genetic technology on an individual level, suggesting that it is acceptable "for couples to make their own attempts to use genetic technologies and knowledge to improve the potential of their offspring." They view it as "the result of individual reproductive choice" and assert that the choice to genetically modify one's unborn children is morally sound if it is not the outcome of societal or institutional coercion. In addition, science correspondent Ronald Bailey insists that choosing genetic enhancement is better than "submitting to the tyranny of chance, which cruelly deals out futures blighted with ill health, stunted mental abilities, and early death."

Nonetheless, many critics of eugenics contend that the use of germline genetic engineering for any purpose would lead to the selective extinction of particular human traits. According to philosophy professor Josep M. Esquirol, even therapeutic germline engineering may threaten society because "the distinction between *improvement towards normality* [through genetics] and the *improvement of normality* is indecisive." Esquirol claims that using genetics to prevent serious conditions will encourage the use of genetics to prevent less serious problems and would ultimately result in genetically enhancing human beings to achieve biological superiority. Others claim that eugenics and genetic enhancement would alienate the biologically flawed members of society. Social commentator Adam Wolfson alleges that "eugenics' unmistakable message to the disabled is this: Better had you never been born. Better had you never burdened society with your deformities."

Germline genetic engineering has yet to be perfected, but discussion of its possible uses in medicine is well under way. In February 2001, draft sequences of the entire human genetic code were made public, linking many diseases and conditions to genetic origins and increasing the hope that prenatal genetic screening and genetic intervention may potentially save future generations from inheritable diseases and conditions. However, the looming history of atrocities committed in the name of eugenics compels others to conclude that using genetic engineering for therapeutic purposes will unavoidably lead to the systematic control of human genetic stock to maintain a genetic standard. *Biomedical Ethics: Opposing Viewpoints* examines the major arguments surrounding genetic engineering and other emerging biomedical technologies in the following chapters: Is Human Cloning Ethical? What Ethics Should Guide Organ Donations? Are Reproductive Technologies Ethical? What Ethics Should Guide Genetic Research? Society's increasing dependence on technology underscores the need to fully understand and carefully consider the implications of these biomedical advances.

CHAPTER 1

Is Human Cloning Ethical?

Chapter Preface

In February 1997, a team of scientists led by embryologist Ian Wilmut announced that they had successfully cloned a sheep named Dolly from the mammary cell of a ewe. Although frogs, insects, and other living creatures had been cloned years earlier, Wilmut and his colleagues were the first to clone an adult mammal, representing an unprecedented breakthrough in cloning technology.

Because of this significant technological advancement, the science fiction scenario of human cloning became a scientific possibility overnight, sparking the race to clone the first human being. In 1997, Clonaid was the first company established to develop safe and reliable human cloning procedures. The year after, physicist Richard Seed claimed that he could clone a human being in less than two years if he had the appropriate resources. In 2001, despite Italy's ban on human cloning experiments, Italian professor Severino Antinori and reproductive specialist Panos Zavos announced that they were commencing attempts to clone humans for infertile couples. In November of the same year, both Clonaid and Advanced Cell Technology, a major biotechnology company, claimed they had successfully cloned human embryos. As of January 2002, further developments regarding these embryos have not been reported.

Although these efforts have not yet produced an actual human being, they have renewed a decades-old debate over the ethics of reproductive human cloning. A major question in this debate is whether human cloning violates the cloned person's individuality. Leon R. Kass, a long-time opponent of human cloning, contends that "a cloned individual—copied from whomever—will be saddled with a genotype that has already lived. He will not be a surprise to the world: people are likely always to compare his doings in life with those of his alter ego."

However, others claim that a cloned human would have as much individuality as anyone else. As stated by biomedical ethicist Rebecca Wynn, "It is unclear why someone who has been cloned will have less autonomy than someone produced by normal sexual reproduction. . . . Whether someone has picked our genotype or not, is simply irrelevant."

In August 2001, the U.S. House of Representatives passed a ban on human cloning. Cloning cannot be used to produce human embryos, whether the intent is to create human life or for the purposes of human embryo experimentation. Nonetheless, as private biotechnology companies continue to advance cloning technology, the human cloning controversy will remain. In the following chapter, the authors discuss the ethical dilemmas of applying this technology to human beings.

"Direct human cloning will be one more option among many specialized medical interventions in human reproduction."

Human Cloning Is Ethical

Nathan Myhrvold

In the following viewpoint, Nathan Myhrvold contends that attacks on the ethics of human cloning are unjustified. The author asserts that human cloning is acceptable because everyone has the right to reproduce and because cloning would be achieved mainly with procedures already used in assisted reproduction. He concludes that the fear of human clones amounts to racism because it is discrimination based on a person's genetic traits. Myhrvold is a quantum physicist and former chief technical officer at Microsoft.

As you read, consider the following questions:
1. According to Myhrvold, what is the infant mortality rate in "truly natural" human reproduction?
2. In the author's view, how is the ethical dilemma of human cloning rooted in jealousy?
3. In Myhrvold's opinion, what benefits may be gained from human cloning research?

If you can clone a sheep, you can almost certainly clone a human being. Some of the most powerful people in the world have felt compelled to act against this threat. President Clinton swiftly imposed a ban on federal funding for human-cloning research. Bills are in the works in both houses of Congress to outlaw human cloning—a step urged on all governments by the pope himself. Cloning humans is taken to be either 1) a fundamentally evil thing that must be stopped or, at the very least, 2) a complex ethical issue that needs legislation and regulation. But what, exactly, is so bad about it?

Start by asking whether human beings have a right to reproduce. I say "yes." I have no moral right to tell other people they shouldn't be able to have children, and I don't see that Bill Clinton has that right either. When Clinton says, "Let us resist the temptation to copy ourselves," it comes from a man not known for resisting other temptations of the flesh. And for a politician, making noise about cloning is pretty close to a fleshly temptation itself. It's an easy way to show sound-bite leadership on an issue that everybody is talking about, without much risk of bitter consequences. After all, how much federally funded research was stopped by this ban? Probably almost none, because Clinton has maintained Ronald Reagan's policy of minimizing federal grants for research in human reproduction. Besides, most researchers thought cloning humans was impossible—so, for the moment, there's unlikely to be a grant-request backlog. There is nothing like banning the nonexistent to show true leadership.

First Century Rules vs. a Twenty-First Century Issue

The pope, unlike the president, is known for resisting temptation. He also openly claims the authority to decide how people reproduce. I respect the pope's freedom to lead his religion, and his followers' freedom to follow his dictate. But calling for secular governments to implement a ban, thus extending his power beyond those he can persuade, shows rather explicitly that the pope does *not* respect the freedom of others. The basic religious doctrine he follows was set down some two millennia ago. Sheep feature prominently in the Bible, but cloning does not. So the pope's views on cloning are 1st century rules applied using 15th century religious thinking to a 21st century issue.

If humans have a right to reproduce, what right does society have to limit the means? Essentially all reproduction is done these days with medical help—at delivery, and often before. Truly natural human reproduction would mean 50 percent infant mortality and make pregnancy-related death the No. 1 killer of adult women.

True, some forms of medical help are more invasive than others. With in vitro fertilization, the sperm and egg are combined in the lab and surgically implanted in the womb. Less than two decades ago, a similar concern was raised over the ethical issues involved in "test-tube babies." To date, nearly 30,000 such babies have been born in the United States alone. Many would-be parents have been made happy. Who has been harmed?

The cloning procedure is similar to IVF. The only difference is that the DNA of sperm and egg would be replaced by DNA from an adult cell. What law or principle—secular, humanist, or religious—says that one combination of genetic material in a flask is OK, but another is not? No matter how closely you study the 1st century texts, I don't think you'll find the answer.

A World of Clones

Even if people have the right to do it, is cloning a good idea? Suppose that every prospective parent in the world stopped having children naturally, and instead produced clones of themselves. What would the world be like in another 20 or 30 years? The answer is: much like today. Cloning would only copy the genetic aspects of people who are already here. Hating a world of clones is hating the current populace. Never before was Pogo so right: We have met the enemy, and he is *us*!

A different scare scenario is a world filled with copies of famous people only. We'll treat celebrity DNA like designer clothes, hankering for Michael Jordan's genes the way we covet his Nike sneakers today. But even celebrity infatuation has its limits. People are not more taken with celebrities than they are with themselves. Besides, such a trend would correct itself in a generation or two, because celebrity is closely linked to rarity. The world seems amused by one Howard Stern, but give us a hundred or a million of them, and they'll seem a lot less endearing.

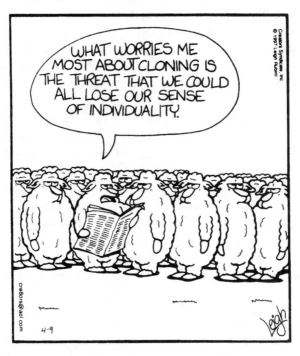

Rubin. © 1997 by Leigh Rubin. Reprinted by permission of the Creators Syndicate.

Clones already exist. About one in every 1,000 births results in a pair of babies with the same DNA. We know them as identical twins. Scientific studies on such twins—reared together or apart—show that they share many characteristics. Just how many they share is a contentious topic in human biology. But genetic determinism is largely irrelevant to the cloning issue. Despite how many or how few individual characteristics twins—or other clones—have in common, *they are different people in the most fundamental sense.* They have their own identities, their own thoughts, and their own rights. Should you be confused on this point, just ask a twin.

Suppose that *Unsolved Mysteries* called you with news of a long-lost identical twin. Would that suddenly make you less of a person, less of an individual? It is hard to see how. So, why would a clone be different? Your clone would be raised in a different era by different people—like the lost identical twin, only younger than you. A person's basic humanity is not governed by how he or she came into this world, or whether somebody else happens to have the same DNA.

Twins aren't the only clones in everyday life. Think about seedless grapes or navel oranges—if there are no seeds, where *did* they come from? It's the plant equivalent of virgin birth—which is to say that they are all clones, propagated by cutting a shoot and planting it. Wine is almost entirely a cloned product. The grapes used for wine have seeds, but they've been cloned from shoots for more than a hundred years in the case of many vineyards. The same is true for many flowers. Go to a garden store, and you'll find products with delightful names like "Olivia's Cloning Compound," a mix of hormones to dunk on the cut end of a shoot to help it take root.

Great Leader, Version 2.0?

One recurring image in anti-cloning propaganda is of some evil dictator raising an army of cloned warriors. Excuse me, but who is going to raise such an army ("raise" in the sense used by parents)? Clones start out life as *babies*. Armies are far easier to raise the old fashioned way—by recruiting or drafting naive young adults. *Dulce et decorum est pro patria mori* ["It is sweet and fitting to die for one's country"] has worked well enough to send countless young men to their deaths through the ages. Why mess with success?

Remember that cloning is not the same as genetic engineering. We don't get to make superman—we have to find him first. Maybe we could clone the superwarrior from Congressional Medal of Honor winners. Their bravery might—or might not—be genetically determined. But, suppose that it is. You might end up with such a brave battalion of heroes that when a grenade lands in their midst, there is a competition to see who gets to jump on it to save the others. Admirable perhaps, but not necessarily the way to win a war. And what about the supply sergeants? The army has a lot more of them than heroes. You could try to breed an expert for every job, including the petty bureaucrats, but what's the point? There's not exactly a shortage of them.

What if Saddam Hussein clones were to rule Iraq for another thousand years? Sounds bad, but Saddam's natural son Uday is reputed to make his father seem saintly by comparison. We have no more to fear from a clone of Saddam, or of Hitler, than we do from their natural-born kin—which is to say, we don't have much to fear: Dictators' kids rarely pose a problem. Stalin's daughter retired to Arizona, and Kim Jong Il of North Korea is laughable as Great Leader, Version 2.0.

The notion of an 80-year-old man cloning himself to cheat death is quaint, but it is unrealistic. First, the baby wouldn't really be him. Second, is the old duffer really up to changing diapers? A persistent octogenarian might convince a younger couple to have his clone and raise it, but that is not much different from fathering a child via a surrogate mother.

Another Form of Racism

Fear of clones is just another form of racism. We all agree it is wrong to discriminate against people based on a set of genetic characteristics known as "race." Calls for a ban on cloning amount to discrimination against people based on another genetic trait—the fact that somebody already has an identical DNA sequence. The most extreme form of discrimination is genocide—seeking to eliminate that which is different. In this case, the genocide is pre-emptive—clones are *so* scary that we must eliminate them before they exist with a ban on their creation.

What is so special about natural reproduction anyway? Cloning is the only predictable way to reproduce, because it creates the identical twin of a known adult. Sexual reproduction is a crap shoot by comparison—some random mix of mom and dad. In evolutionary theory, this combination is thought to help stir the gene pool, so to speak. However, evolution for humans is essentially over, because we use medical science to control the death rate.

Whatever the temptations of cloning, the process of natural reproduction will always remain a *lot* more fun. An expensive and uncomfortable lab procedure will never offer any real competition for sex. The people most likely to clone will be those in special circumstances—infertile couples who must endure IVF anyway, for example. Even there, many will mix genetics to mimic nature. Another special case is where one member of a couple has a severe genetic disease. They might choose a clone of the healthy parent, rather than burden their child with a joint heritage that could be fatal.

The most upsetting possibility in human cloning isn't superwarriors or dictators. It's that rich people with big egos will clone themselves. The common practice of giving a boy the same name as his father or choosing a family name for a child of either sex reflects our hunger for vicarious immortality. Clones may resonate with this instinct and cause some people to reproduce this way. So what? Rich and egotistic folks do all sorts of annoying things, and the law is hardly the means with which to try and stop them.

The "deep ethical issues" about cloning mainly boil down to jealousy. Economic jealousy is bad enough, and it is a factor here, but the thing that truly drives people crazy is sexual jealousy. Eons of evolution through sexual selection have made the average man or woman insanely jealous of any interloper who gains a reproductive advantage—say by diddling your spouse. Cloning is less personal than cuckoldry, but it strikes a similar chord: Someone has got the reproductive edge on you.

The Fruits of Science

Once the fuss has died down and further animal research has paved the way, direct human cloning will be one more option among many specialized medical interventions in human reproduction, affecting only a tiny fraction of the population. Research into this area could bring far wider benefits. Clinton's knee-jerk policy changes nothing in the short run, but it is ultimately a giant step backward. In using an adult cell to create a clone, the "cellular clock" that determines the difference between an embryo and adult was somehow reset. Work in this area might help elucidate the process by which aging occurs and yield a way to reset the clocks in some of our own cells, allowing us to regenerate. Selfishly speaking, that would be more exciting to me than cloning, because it would help *me*. That's a lot more directly useful than letting me sire an identical twin 40 years my junior.

To some, the scientist laboring away to unlock the mysteries of life is a source of evil, never to be trusted. To others, including me, the scientist is the ray of light, illuminating the processes that make the universe work and making us better through that knowledge. Various arguments can be advanced toward either view, but one key statistic is squarely on my side. The vast majority of people, including those who rail against science, owe their very lives to previous medical discoveries. They embody the fruits of science. Don't let the forces of darkness, ignorance, and fear turn us back from research. Instead, let us raise—and yes, even clone—new generations of hapless ingrates, who can whine and rail against the discoveries of the next age.

"In cloning technologies we may face the highest price of all: the end of the perception of human life as 'sacred.'"

Human Cloning Is Unethical

Wesley J. Smith

Wesley J. Smith is an attorney for the International Anti-Euthanasia Task Force and author of The Culture of Death: The Assault on Medical Ethics in America. In the following viewpoint, Smith opposes human cloning on the grounds that it will lead to eugenics—the genetic engineering of human beings in order to perpetuate desirable traits and eliminate flaws among the species. He argues that human cloning is an attempt to control the fate of human evolution, which would undermine the intrinsic worth and equality of all individuals.

As you read, consider the following questions:
1. In the author's view, what is the sanctity of life ethic?
2. In Smith's opinion, how are cloning advocates similar to eugenicists of the mid–twentieth century?
3. According to Smith, what are human/animal chimeras?

Excerpted from "Cloning Reality," by Wesley J. Smith, *Mindszenty Report*, v. XLIII, February 2001. Copyright © 2001 by the Mindszenty Report. Reprinted with permission.

B rave New World has arrived at last, as we always knew it would. On January 22, 2001, Britain's House of Lords voted overwhelmingly to permit the cloning and maintenance of human embryos up to 14 days old for the purposes of medical experimentation, thereby taking the first terrible step toward the legalization of full-blown human cloning. Meanwhile, an international group of human-reproduction experts announced their plans—current legal prohibitions be damned—to bring cloned humans to birth in order to provide biological children to infertile couples. They expect to deliver their first clone within 18 months. The ripple effect on human history of these and the events that will inevitably follow may well make a tsunami seem like a mere splash in a playground puddle.

Human cloning is moving slowly but surely toward reality despite intense and widespread opposition throughout the world. Many resisters worry that permitting human cloning would remove us from the natural order. As the venerable [medical ethics professor] Leon R. Kass has so eloquently put it, cloning brings conception and gestation "into the bright light of the laboratory, beneath which the child-to-be can be fertilized, nourished, pruned, weeded, watched, inspected, prodded, pinched, cajoled, injected, tested, rated, graded, approved, stamped, wrapped, sealed, and delivered."

Kass's point is that once human life is special-ordered rather than conceived, life will never be the same. No longer will each of us be a life that is unique from all others who have ever lived. Instead our genetic selves will be molded and chiseled in a Petri dish to comply with the social norms of the day. And if something goes wrong, the new life will be thrown away like some defective widget or other fungible product. So long, diversity. Hello homogeneity.

Cloning Versus Sanctity of Life

Perhaps even worse, widespread acceptance of cloning would be a deathblow to the sanctity/equality of life ethic—the cornerstone of Western liberty from which sprang our still unrealized dream of universal human rights. The premise of the sanctity of life ethic is that each and every one of us is of equal, incalculable, moral worth. Whatever our race, sex, ethnicity, stature, health, disability, age, beauty, or cognitive capacity, we are all full moral equals within the human community—there is no "them," only "us."

Cloning stands in stark opposition to this equalitarian dream. It is—and always has been—the quintessential eugenic enterprise.

Eugenics, meaning "good in birth," directly contradicts the self-evident truth enunciated by Thomas Jefferson that all people are created equal. Eugenicists believe that the moral value of people is relative, or to put it another way, that some of us are better than others of us. Eugenicists seek to "improve" humanity by breeding out the "undesirable" traits of those deemed less worthy.

Indeed, the pioneers of the eugenics movement worked for more than 50 years during the late 1800s and into the middle of the 20th Century to eliminate the genes of the "unfit" from the human genome, first by encouraging proper eugenic marriages (positive eugenics) and more perniciously, by involuntarily sterilizing those deemed to have undesirable physical and personal traits (negative eugenics).

Directing Evolution

Anyone with even a modicum of historical knowledge—alas, a scarce commodity in these post-modernistic times—knows where that led. In this country alone, 60,000-plus people were involuntarily sterilized. In Western Europe, eugenics belief systems combusted with social Darwinism and anti-Semitism to produce the Nazis and thence to the Holocaust.

Today's eugenicists are not racist or anti-Semites but they exhibit every bit as much hubris as their predecessors by assuming that they—that we—have the right to direct the future evolution of humanity, only now rather than having to rely on clunky procreative planning they literally grasp the human genome in their hands. Cloning plays a big part in these plans as the patriarch of the modern bioethics movement, Joseph Fletcher, a wild eugenicist, well knew when he wrote nearly 30 years ago that cloning would "permit the preservation and perpetuation of the finest genotypes that arise in our species."

What are these supposedly "finest" genotypes? Most neoeugenicist cloning advocates worship at the altar of the frontal lobe, valuing high intelligence and logical thinking in much the same way that founding practitioners of eugenics valued the blue eyes and blond hair they saw each morning in their own mirrors.

Issues of Identity

Cloning creates serious issues of identity and individuality. The cloned person may experience concerns about his distinctive identity not only because he will be in genotype and appearance identical to another human being, but, in this case, because he may also be twin to the person who is his "father" or "mother"—if one can still call them that. What would be the psychic burdens of being the "child" or "parent" of your twin?

Leon Kass, *The Ethics of Human Cloning*, 1998.

Thus, Princeton University's Lee Silver hopes through cloning to create a "special group of mental beings" who "will be as different from humans as humans are from the primitive worms . . . that first crawled along the earth's surface." Yet Fletcher, Silver, and most others of their ilk almost always miss the point that smart people are not necessarily good people. And they rarely discuss designing people with the most important human capacities of all: the ability to love unconditionally, gentleness, empathy, the deep desire to be helpful and productive. Ironically, these highest, best human characteristics are often found in people with Down's syndrome or other developmental disabilities—the very people who the neo-eugenicists believe should be evolved intentionally out of existence whether through genetic manipulation or if necessary, selective abortion and infanticide.

Playing God

Eugenics, as awful as it is, is only the beginning of the threat posed to the natural order by human cloning. Some cloners have decided that if they are going to "play God"; they might as well do it all the way by creating altogether new life forms. Indeed, scientists have already used cloning techniques to add jellyfish genetic material to a cloned monkey embryo, manufacturing a monkey that glows in the dark. Nor is human life itself immune from such "Dr. Moreau" forms of manipulation. For example, some in bioethics and bioscience support the creation of chimeras—part human and part animal—beings Joseph Fletcher called "parahumans" who he hoped would be "fashioned to do dangerous and demeaning jobs."

In other words, Fletcher advocated the creation of a slave race of mostly-humans designed by us and for our use. "As it is now," the bioethics patriarch wrote in his typically snobbish fashion, "low grade work is shoved off on moronic and retarded individuals, the victims of uncontrolled reproduction. Should we not program such workers 'thoughtfully' instead of accidentally, by means of hybridization?"

Fletcher's dark dream of human/animal chimeras is well on its way to reality. Not too long ago Australian scientists announced they had created a "pig-man" through cloning techniques, and allowed the hybrid to develop for more than two weeks before destroying it. Last year, a biotech company took out a Europe-wide patent on embryos containing cells both from humans and from mice, sheep, pigs, cattle, goats, or fish. Where such manipulations will lead may be beyond comprehension.

Cloning presents humankind with the postmodernist version of the Faustian bargain. Through cloning, we are told, our greatest dreams can be realized: the barren can give birth, genetic anomalies and disabilities can be eliminated at the embryonic level, near immortality will be within our grasp as replacements, for worn out organs can be grown in the lab for transplantation without fear of bodily rejection. But the devil always demands his due—the higher the "value" of the bargain, the greater the price.

In cloning technologies we may face the highest price of all: the end of the perception of human life as "sacred" and the concomitant increase in the nihilistic belief that humans are mere biological life; an increasing willingness to use and exploit human life as if it were a mere national resource; eventually, the loss of human diversity itself—and these are just the foreseen consequences. The unforeseen consequences of mucking around in the human genome may be worse than we can imagine. As Leon Kass has written, "shallow are the souls that have forgotten how to shudder."

| *"Cloning research must be allowed to continue . . . because it entails benefits that should not be scrapped outright because of perceived risks."*

Cloning Technology Could Be Beneficial to Humans

Part I: Michel Revel; Part II: Human Cloning Foundation

In the following two-part viewpoint, genetics professor Michel Revel and the Human Cloning Foundation (HCF) contend that cloning technology may yield greater benefits than risks to humans. In Part I, Michel Revel maintains that halting human cloning research before discovering its full potential may come at a great cost to scientific discovery. Revel concludes that human cloning research should be allowed within ethical guidelines that consider the benefits, risks, and rights of individuals. In Part II, the HCF describes specific ways in which cloning technology may benefit society. Revel is a member of the United Nations Educational, Scientific, and Cultural Organization (UNESCO). The HCF (www.humancloning.org) is a nonprofit website that supports human cloning and its technologies.

As you read, consider the following questions:
1. What are Revel's views of reproduction by human cloning?
2. What differing views of embryonic life does Revel describe?
3. Why does the HCF support the cloning of a dead child?

Part I: From "Outright Condemnation of Cloning Research Is Premature," by Michel Revel, *The Scientist*, January 19, 1998. Copyright © 1998 by The Scientist, Inc. Reprinted with permission. Part II: Excerpted from "The Benefits of Human Cloning," by the Human Cloning Foundation, www.humancloning.org, July 19, 2001. Copyright © 1998 by the Human Cloning Foundation. Reprinted with permission.

I

"The more knowledge, the more distress," says the Talmud. How true that seems for the field of genetics. As soon as advances in laboratory animals are announced, the news is used to forecast a revolution in human reproduction: Let's make genetically ideal babies, let's clone human copies, let's make headless fetuses for transplantable spare parts.

A Convenient Target

Biology has become a convenient target for moralists and politicians who condemn science and are eager to ban new experimentation. "To benefit from scientific advancement" is a basic human right defined by the United Nations. Exercising this right implies defining the limits of the permissible and weighing the moral conditions of action. Ethics committees ought to explain the potential benefits of scientific applications and create guidelines for their use, rather than try to have them outlawed up front.

Fear of eugenics and of illusory social manipulations has led several governments to outlaw applications of cloning to humans. In a revised text of its Universal Declaration on the Human Genome and Human Rights adopted at the organization's General Conference on November 12, the United Nations Educational, Scientific, and Cultural Organization (UNESCO) added a statement defining cloning as "contrary to human dignity."

I believe that one could have adopted another position. Indeed, ethicists who drafted the original UNESCO declaration meant to ensure that application of any genetic practice to human beings be developed with respect for the rights and dignity of individuals. They also meant to ensure that mankind would not be deprived of benefits such progress might bring if applied within the bioethical guidelines outlined eloquently in the rest of the declaration. For these reasons, several delegations proposed not to rush in condemning any particular technique, including cloning.

Reproduction by Cloning

It may be worth remembering that after the first human *in vitro* fertilization in 1978, "creating a human being in a test

31

tube" was criticized as undignified and offensive to human love. Since then, assisted reproduction has alleviated distress for thousands of parents. Speculating that it may one day be safely achieved, cloning could be just another form of assisted reproduction. Fertilization by an adult cell nucleus—the essence of cloning—may be invaluable for a man and a woman who are both sterile and desire a biological child, or a religious couple who consider an extramaritally donated sperm or egg adulterous.

Reproduction by cloning may also hold a solution when one partner carries a severe hereditary disease, allowing the other partner to contribute his or her genome to their offspring. This is why some countries, including Israel, consider it sufficient to strictly regulate rather than ban cloning research.

Hoping to make an exact replica of oneself by cloning is unrealistic. Cloned human beings would resemble each other no more than monozygotic twins. Cognitive abilities are patterned by education and environment as well as genetics. Genetic identity is an illusion; cloned animals differ in their hair color patterns. The immune system of each human being is different, and so may be brain wiring. The surrogate egg and its mitochondrial DNA exert a maternal influence on the development, as does the pregnant mother's nutritional behavior. Obviously, there can be no substitute for mixing human genes through sexual reproduction and for the diversity that underlies the unity of the human species. The key to avoiding megalomaniac attempts to improve racial human subgroups or produce human beings with "useful traits" is to ensure that the technology serves only the needs of the individual and not goals desired by society. It must never be used except for therapeutic purposes, respecting the rights, autonomy, and dignity of the mother, of the donor, and of the child to be born. The rights and wrongs of any genetic manipulation should be decided on a case-by-case basis.

Research Should Not Be Scrapped

Cloning research must be allowed to continue within agreed guidelines because it entails benefits that should not be scrapped outright because of perceived risks. Cloning may help overcome present hazards of graft procedures. Embryonic cells could be taken from cloned embryos prior to implantation into the uterus and cultured to form tissues of pancreatic cells to treat diabetes, or brain nerve cells that could be genetically engineered to treat Parkinson's or other neurodegenerative diseases.

Genetically Safer

The first argument raised by those who fear cloning is that it would create monsters, genetic mistakes that are stillborn or, even worse, that survive to birth. How could we risk such a disaster? critics ask. But, [scientist Lee] Silver replies, cloning is actually genetically safer than normal sexual reproduction because it bypasses the most common form of birth defect—having the wrong number of chromosomes. . . .

The chromosomal abnormalities occur when sperm and egg cells are produced. In the testes of a man and in the ovaries of a woman, progenitors of sperm and egg cells mature. As they do so, they divide repeatedly and develop into cells that have a single copy of each chromosome instead of the usual two copies. When that happens, some sperm and some eggs accidentally end up with one chromosome too many or one chromosome too few.

With cloning, such chromosome mixups cannot occur, Silver pointed out. After all, you are starting with a normal cell, from a normal adult, with the proper number of chromosomes. So the major cause of birth defects is ruled out.

Gina Kolata, *Clone: The Road to Dolly and the Path Ahead*, 1998.

Whether producing embryos for such purposes is ethical will depend on views toward early embryonic life, as well as on whether saving an existing human life justifies ending that of embryos. Christianity sanctifies life from fertilization, while Judaism and Islam consider the embryo to acquire human characteristics only after 40 days. Scientific guidelines allow embryos to be grown in culture for 14 days. The ethical discussion should respect individual religions and philosophies.

The lack of consensus on what makes an embryo into a human being will affect the debate on headless embryos that could provide formed organs for grafts. Lethal fetal malformations have been recognized since antiquity, and moralists have considered fetuses with no identifiable head and chest as nonhumans. Whether saving a human life by willfully producing such fetal abortuses is compatible with human dignity will be debated—and ought to be—considering that a woman will have to bear the fetus. At the same time, the unavailability of organs is becoming a major death factor that will worsen unless scientists successfully culture fully formed organs. Today's organ traffic could appear to many a more dangerous peril than producing one's own cloned embryo for autograft.

Ethics should weigh the rights of the individual to benefit from scientific advancement against the risks, and strictly regulate or sometimes delay rather than condemn. Demonization of science and up front banning of potential new technologies is not a dignified human answer.

II

There are many ways in which human cloning is expected to benefit mankind. Below is a list that is far from complete.

• *Rejuvenation.* Dr. Richard Seed, one of the leading proponents of human cloning technology, suggests that it may someday be possible to reverse the aging process because of what we learn from cloning.

• *Human cloning technology could be used to reverse heart attacks.* Scientists believe that they may be able to treat heart attack victims by cloning their healthy heart cells and injecting them into the areas of the heart that have been damaged. Heart disease is the number one killer in the United States and several other industrialized countries.

• *There has been a breakthrough with human stem cells.* Embryonic stem cells can be grown to produce organs or tissues to repair or replace damaged ones. Skin for burn victims, brain cells for the brain damaged, spinal cord cells for quadriplegics and paraplegics, hearts, lungs, livers, and kidneys could be produced. By combining this technology with human cloning technology it may be possible to produce needed tissue for suffering people that will be free of rejection by their immune systems. Conditions such as Alzheimer's disease, Parkinson's disease, diabetes, heart failure, degenerative joint disease, and other problems may be made curable if human cloning and its technology are not banned.

• *Infertility.* With cloning, infertile couples could have children. Despite getting a fair amount of publicity in the news current treatments for infertility, in terms of percentages, are not very successful. One estimate is that current infertility treatments are less than 10 percent successful. Couples go through physically and emotionally painful procedures for a small chance of having children. Many couples run out of time and money without successfully having children. Human cloning could make it possible for many more infertile couples to have children than ever before possible.

• *Plastic, reconstructive, and cosmetic surgery.* Because of human cloning and its technology, the days of silicone breast implants and other cosmetic procedures that may cause immune disease should soon be over. With the new technology, instead of using materials foreign to the body for such procedures, doctors will be able to manufacture bone, fat, connective tissue, or cartilage that matches the patients' tissues exactly. Anyone will be able to have their appearance altered to their satisfaction without the leaking of silicone gel into their bodies or the other problems that occur with present-day plastic surgery. Victims of terrible accidents that deform the face should now be able to have their features repaired with new, safer technology. Limbs for amputees may be able to be regenerated.

• *Breast implants.* Most people are aware of the breast implant fiasco in which hundreds of thousands of women received silicone breast implants for cosmetic reasons. Many came to believe that the implants were making them ill with diseases of their immune systems. With human cloning and its technology breast augmentation and other forms of cosmetic surgery could be done with implants that would not be any different from the person's normal tissues.

• *Defective genes.* The average person carries 8 defective genes inside them. These defective genes allow people to become sick when they would otherwise remain healthy. With human cloning and its technology it may be possible to ensure that we no longer suffer because of our defective genes.

• *Down's syndrome.* Those women at high risk for Down's syndrome can avoid that risk by cloning.

• *Tay-Sachs disease.* This autosomal recessive genetic disorder could be prevented by using cloning to ensure that a child does not express the gene for the disorder.

- *Liver failure*. We may be able to clone livers for liver transplants.
- *Kidney failure*. We may be able to clone kidneys for kidney transplants.
- *Leukemia*. We should be able to clone the bone marrow for children and adults suffering from leukemia. This is expected to be one of the first benefits to come from cloning technology.
- *Cancer*. We may learn how to switch cells on and off through cloning and thus be able to cure cancer. Scientists still do not know exactly how cells differentiate into specific kinds of tissue, nor do they understand why cancerous cells lose their differentiation. Cloning, at long last, may be the key to understanding differentiation and cancer.
- *Cystic fibrosis*. We may be able to produce effective genetic therapy against cystic fibrosis. Ian Wilmut and colleagues are already working on this problem.
- *Spinal cord injury*. We may learn to grow nerves or the spinal cord back again when they are injured. Quadriplegics might be able to get out of their wheelchairs and walk again. Christopher Reeve, the man who played Superman, might be able to walk again.
- *Testing for genetic disease*. Cloning technology can be used to test for and perhaps cure genetic diseases.

Unparalleled Advancement

The above list only scratches the surface of what human cloning technology can do for mankind. The suffering that can be relieved is staggering. This new technology heralds a new era of unparalleled advancement in medicine if people will release their fears and let the benefits begin. Why should another child die from leukemia when, if the technology is allowed, we should be able to cure it in a few years' time?

From e-mail to the Human Cloning Foundation it is clear that many people would support human cloning in the following situations:

1) A couple has one child then they become infertile and cannot have more children. Cloning would enable such a couple to have a second child, perhaps a younger twin of the child they already have.

2) A child is lost soon after birth to a tragic accident. Many parents have written the HCF after losing a baby in a fire, car accident, or other unavoidable disaster. These grief-stricken parents often say that they would like to have their perfect baby back. Human cloning would allow such parents to have a twin of their lost baby, but it would be like other twins, a unique individual and not a carbon copy of the child that was lost under heartbreaking circumstances.

3) A woman who through some medical emergency ended up having a hysterectomy before being married or having children. Such women have been stripped of their ability to have children. These women need a surrogate mother to have a child of their own DNA, which can be done either by human cloning or by in vitro fertilization.

4) A boy graduates from high school at age 18. He goes to a pool party to celebrate. He confuses the deep end and shallow end and dives head first into the pool, breaking his neck and becoming a quadriplegic. At age 19 he has his first urinary tract infection because of an indwelling urinary catheter and continues to suffer from them the rest of his life. At age 20 he comes down with herpes zoster of the trigeminal nerve. He suffers chronic unbearable pain. At age 21 he inherits a 10 million dollar trust fund. He never marries or has children. At age 40 after hearing about Dolly being a clone, he changes his will and has his DNA stored for future human cloning. His future mother will be awarded one million dollars to have him and raise him. His DNA clone will inherit a trust fund. He leaves five million to spinal cord research. He dies feeling that although he was robbed of normal life, his twin/clone will lead a better life.

5) Two parents have a baby boy. Unfortunately the baby has muscular dystrophy. They have another child and it's another boy with muscular dystrophy. They decide not to have any more children. Each boy has over 20 operations as doctors attempt to keep them healthy and mobile. Both boys die as teenagers. The childless parents donate their estate to curing muscular dystrophy and to having their boys cloned when medical science advances enough so that their DNA can live again, but free of muscular dystrophy.

> *"To allow [human] cloning is to open the door to a scarier enterprise: genetically engineering people without their consent."*

Cloning Technology Would Not Benefit Humans

John F. Kilner

John F. Kilner is the executive director of the Center for Bioethics and Human Dignity in Bannockburn, Illinois. In the following viewpoint, Kilner argues that the potential social risks of human cloning are greater than its medical benefits. He warns that allowing human cloning would permit the genetic engineering of people to suit societal purposes. In addition, Kilner claims that there are alternative ways to achieve the medical benefits promised by human cloning technology.

As you read, consider the following questions:
1. In the author's opinion, how does the film *Multiplicity* contribute to misunderstanding about cloning?
2. According to Kilner, which potential uses for cloning would "demean" humans?
3. In Kilner's view, how may emphasis upon cloning research harm other fields of medicine?

Excerpted from "Human Cloning," by John F. Kilner, *Physician*, www.family.org/physmag, July 19, 2001. Copyright © 2000 by Physician Magazine. Reprinted with permission.

We live in a brave new world in which reproductive technologies are ravaging as well as replenishing families. The new eugenics is simply the latest version of the age-old quest to make human beings—in fact, humanity as a whole—the way we want them to be. It includes our efforts to be rid of unwanted human beings through abortion and euthanasia. It more recently is focusing on our growing ability to understand and manipulate our genetic code, which directs the formation of many aspects of who we are, for better and for worse.

We aspire to complete control over the code, though at this point relatively little control is possible. Yet it is this backdrop that can help us understand the great fascination with human cloning today, which promises to give us a substantial measure of control over the genetic make-up of our offspring. We cannot control their code exactly, but the first major step in that direction is hugely appealing: You can have a child whose genetic code is virtually identical to your own. *And you didn't turn out so badly, did you?!*

Admittedly, in our most honest moments we would improve a few things about ourselves. So the larger agenda here remains complete genetic control. But human cloning represents one concrete step in that direction, and the forces pushing us from behind to take that step are tremendous. Sheep and other animals have been cloned, though the latest sheep research suggests that the clones are not truly identical to the originals. So we can expect human cloning to be alluringly close at hand. If we have any serious qualms about human cloning, we need to voice them now, in publicly understandable terms, while society is in the process of deciding whether to ban or limit this practice.

What's the Fascination?

Why would people want to clone humans in the first place? Most people respond to the prospect of human cloning in two ways simultaneously: They are deeply squeamish about the idea, and yet they also find something extremely captivating about it. Such fascination is captured in a variety of films, including *The Boys From Brazil* (portraying the attempt to clone the powerful Adolf Hitler), *Bladerunner* (questioning whether a clone would be more like a person or a machine), and *Multiplicity* (presenting a man's attempt to have enough time for his family, job and other pursuits by producing several live adult replicas of himself). Popular discussions ponder the wonderful prospects of creating multiple Mother Teresas, Michael Jordans or whomever.

The greatest problem with creative, media-driven discussions like these is that they often reflect a misunderstanding of the science and people involved. *Multiplicity* presents human replicas, not clones in the form that we are discussing them here. When an adult is cloned (e.g., the adult sheep from which Dolly was cloned), an embryo is created—not another adult. Although the embryo's cells contain the same genetic code as the cells of the adult being cloned, the embryo must go through many years of development in an environment that is significantly different from that in which the adult developed. Because both our environment and our genetics substantially influence who we are, the embryo will not become the same person as the adult. In fact, because people also have a spiritual capacity to evaluate and alter either or both our environment and our genetics, human clones are bound to be quite different from the adults who provide their genetic code.

Weighing the Benefits

Are there any more thoughtful ethical justifications for human cloning? Indeed, many have been put forward, and they most frequently appeal to its utility or benefit. As long as cloning will produce a net increase in human well-being, the rationale goes, it is warranted. People are well-acquainted with the notion of assessing costs and benefits, and it is common to hear the argument that something will produce so much benefit that efforts to block it must surely be misguided. Such justifications for human cloning include the benefits of replacing a dying child with a genetically identical new one and producing a clone of a sick child to provide bone marrow or organs for transplant.

However, there are serious problems with this type of justification. Most significantly, it is unworkable, because knowing with any precision the utility achieved from cloning or any other practice is simply impossible—and it is dangerous. We cannot know all of the ways a practice will affect the people in the world. For example, it is inconceivable that we could accurately quantify the satisfaction of every parent in future centuries who will choose cloning rather than traditional sexual reproduction in order to spare their children from newly discovered genetic problems. In fact, as Ian Wilmut observed shortly after announcing his cloning of Dolly, "Most of the things cloning will be used for have yet to be imagined." The difficulty of comparing the significance of every foreseeable consequence on the same scale of value, including comparing each person's subjective experiences with everyone else's, only adds to the unworkability.

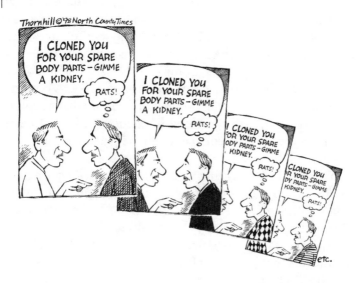

Thornhill. © 1998 by *North County Times*. Reprinted with permission.

In real life, decision-makers intuitively compare only the consequences of which they are most aware and concerned. Such an approach invites bias and discrimination, intended and unintended. Even more dangerous is the absence of limits to what can be justified. There are no built-in protections for weak individuals or minority groups, including clones. People can be subjected to anything—the worst possible oppression or even death—if it is beneficial to the majority. Situations such as Nazi Germany and U.S. slavery can be justified using this way of thinking.

Expendable Beings?

When utility is our basis for justifying what is allowed in society, people are used as mere means to achieve the ends of other people. It may be appropriate to use plants and animals in this way, within limits, but that is another debate. Accordingly, most people do not find it objectionable to clone animals and plants to achieve products that will fulfill a purpose—such as better milk or better grain.

It is demeaning, however, to produce clones simply to provide spare parts, such as vital transplantable organs, for other people. Such cloning fails to respect the equal and great dignity of all people by making some, in effect, the slaves of others. Even cloning a child who dies to remove the parents' grief forces the clone to permanently be subjected to the parents' will. The irony of this last situation? The clone will not become the same child as was lost, as both the child and the clone are the product of far more than their genetics. Not only will the clone be demeaned by not being fully respected and accepted as a unique person, but the parents will fail to regain their lost child in the process.

In other words, showing that a good benefit—even a great benefit—will result is not a sufficient argument to justify an action. Although it is easy to forget this basic point when enticed by the promise of a wonderful benefit, we intuitively know it is true. We recognize that we could, for example, cut up one person, take her or his various organs for transplant, and save many lives as a result. But we do not go around doing that. We realize that if the action we take to achieve the benefit is itself horrendous, beneficial results are not enough to justify it.

Truth and Consequences

To justify human cloning by utility, all the consequences of allowing this practice have to be considered—not just the benefits generated by the exceptional situations commonly cited in its defense. What are some of the consequences we need to be concerned about? There is space here to note only two of the many that weigh heavily against human cloning.

First, as suggested earlier, to allow cloning is to open the door to a scarier enterprise: genetically engineering people without their consent—not for their own benefit, but for the benefit of particular people or society at large. Cloning entails producing a person with a particular genetic code because of the attractiveness or usefulness of a person with that code. In this sense, cloning is just the tip of a much larger genetic iceberg. We are developing the genetic understanding and capability to shape the human genetic code in many ways. If we allow cloning, we legitimate in principle the entire enterprise of designing children to suit parental or social purposes. As one researcher at the U.S. Council on Foreign Relations commented, "Dolly is best understood as a drop in a towering wave [of genetic research] that is about to crash over us." The personal and social destructiveness of large-scale eugenic efforts (including, but by no means limited to, Nazi Germany's) has been substantial, but at least it has been limited to date by our limited genetic understanding and technology. Today the stakes are much higher.

The second critical consideration that must be included in any honest utilitarian calculus involves the allocation of limited resources. To spend resources on the development and practice of human cloning is to not spend them on other endeavors that would be more beneficial to society. For many years now there have been extensive discussions about the rising costs of health care and the huge number of people (tens of millions) even in the United States that do not have health insurance. It has also long been established that such lack of insurance means that significant numbers of people are actually going without necessary health care and are seriously suffering or dying as a result. Inadequate funding yields serious health consequences because there is no alternative way to produce the basic health result at issue.

Not only are the benefits of human cloning less significant than those that could be achieved by expending the same funds on other health care initiatives, but there are alternative ways of bringing children into the world that can yield at least one major benefit of cloning—children themselves. If there were enough resources available to fund every technology needed or wanted by anyone, the situation would be different. But researching and practicing human cloning will result in serious suffering and even loss of life because other pressing health-care needs cannot be met.

Needless to say, it is possible to express our concerns about cloning in theological terms. Bottom line: Using other people without their consent for our ends is a violation of their status as beings created in the image of God. All people have a God-given dignity that prevents us from using them as mere means to achieve our purposes. Knowing that people are created in the image of God (Genesis 1:26–27), biblical writers in both the Old and New Testaments periodically invoke this truth about human beings to argue that people should not be demeaned in various ways (Genesis 9:6; James 3:9).

Claims about utility, then, are woefully inadequate to justify human cloning. In fact, a careful look at utilitarian justifications shows that they provide compelling reasons instead to reject human cloning. To stand up and say so may become more and more risky in our brave new world. As the culture increasingly embraces utilitarian thinking, it will take courage to insist in the new context of cloning that such thinking is inadequate and dangerous. But such a brave new world, echoing the Word of old, is one where we must be bold to speak.

"*Poorly constructed legislation, designed to prohibit the cloning of a human being, could inadvertently interfere with . . . applications of the technologies in medicine.*"

Therapeutic Human Cloning Should Be Permitted

Michael D. West

Some scientists report that embryonic stem cells have the potential to generate all types of human tissues for replacement. Although these cells can be harvested from embryos left over from infertility treatments, stem cell treatment is not used because of the high probability that the body will reject transplanted tissues. In the following viewpoint, Michael D. West claims that therapeutic human cloning—in which embryos are cloned from a patient's own cells—could be a major advance in stem cell treatment. West insists that tissues created from a patient's own embryonic stem cells will not be rejected by their immune system. While he opposes reproductive human cloning, he asserts that research into therapeutic human cloning should be allowed to continue. West is president and chief executive officer of Advanced Cell Technology, a biotechnology company based in Worcester, Massachusetts.

As you read, consider the following questions:
1. In West's opinion, how is the growing aging population affecting health care in the United States?
2. According to the author, how are "totipotent" stem cells different from "pluripotent" stem cells?
3. In West's view, what possible source of oocytes, or eggs, may be used for therapeutic human cloning in the future?

Excerpted from Michael D. West's testimony before the Congressional Science, Technology, and Space Subcommittee on Labor, Health, and Human Services and Education, December 2, 1998.

W e are approaching a period in our national history of unparalleled growth of the elderly sector of the population. The aging of the baby boom population along with a general increase in the number of aged people is expected to increase the number of the elderly sevenfold between 1980 and 2030 A.D. And since the aged use a disproportionately high percentage of health care, this "graying of America" is likely to greatly strain our national resources. It has been estimated that transplantation procedures currently account for nearly half of our health care expenditures, approaching $400 billion annually. This is likely to grow even larger with the aging of our population and result in a marked increase in the demand for transplantation. The increased incidence of age-related degenerative disease will likely lead to conflicts of economics, ethics, and aesthetics as we struggle to find a humane and practical means of treating the ailing. Concrete examples of tissues needed will likely include: heart tissue for heart failure, arrhythmias, and ischemic damage, cartilage for arthritis, neurons for Parkinson's disease, kidney cells for kidney failure, liver cells for cirrhosis and hepatitis, skin for burns and ulcers, and bone marrow transplantations for cancer to name only a few. While current procedures are partially successful in alleviating human suffering, these procedures are limited by two major difficulties: 1) the availability of the needed cell or tissue type, and 2) the histocompatibility of the transplanted tissues. [This refers to the compatibility of transplanted tissues within the human body; a major challenge to the success of organ transplantation.] As a result, thousands of patients die every year for the lack of transplantable cells and tissues and projections from the Bureau of the Census suggest this shortage will worsen with the aging of our population.

Human ES Cells

Human ES cell technologies may greatly improve the availability of diverse cell types. Human ES cells are unique in that they stand near the base of the developmental tree. These cells are frequently designated "totipotent" stem cells, meaning that they are potentially capable of forming any cell or tissue type needed in medicine. These differ from previously isolated stem cells that are "pluripotent" that is, capable of forming several, but only a limited number, of cell types. An example of pluripotent stem cells are the bone marrow stem cells now widely used in the treatment of cancer and other life-threatening diseases.

With appropriate funding of research, we may soon learn to direct these cells to become vehicles of lifesaving potential. We may, for instance, become able to produce neurons for the treatment of Parkinson's disease and spinal cord injury, heart muscle cells for heart failure, cartilage for arthritis and many others as well. This research has great potential to help solve the first problem of tissue availability, but the technologies to direct these cells to become various cell types in adequate quantities remains to be elucidated. Because literally hundreds of cell types are needed, thousands of academic research projects need to be funded, far exceeding the resources of the biotechnology industry.

Seriousness of the Shortage

As promising as ES cell technology may be, it does not solve the second problem of histocompatibility. Human ES cells obtained from embryos derived during in vitro fertilization procedures, or from fetal sources, are essentially cells from another individual (allogeneic). Several approaches can be envisioned to solve the problem of histocompatibility. One approach would be to make vast numbers of human ES cell lines that could be stored in a frozen state. This "library" of cells would then offer varied surface antigens, such that the patient's physician could search through the library for cells that are as close as possible to the patient. But these would likely still require simultaneous immunosuppression that is not always effective. In addition, immunosuppresive therapy carries with it increased cost, and the risk of complications including malignancy and even death.

Another theoretical solution would be to genetically modify the cultured ES cells to make them "universal donor" cells. That is, the cells would have genes added or genes removed that would "mask" the foreign nature of the cells, allowing the patient's immune system to see the cells as "self." While such technologies may be developed in the future, it is also possible that these technologies may carry with them unacceptably high risks of rejection or other complications that would limit their practical utility in clinical practice.

Given the seriousness of the current shortage of transplantable cells and tissues, the FDA has demonstrated a willingness to consider a broad array of options including the sourcing of cells and indeed whole organs from animals (xenografts) although these sources also pose unique problems of histocompatibility. These animal cells do have the advantage that they have the potential to be genetically engineered to approach the status of "universal donor" cells, through genetic engineering. However as described above, no simple procedure to confer such universal donor status is known. Most such procedures are still experimental and would likely continue to require the use of drugs to hold off rejection, drugs that add to health care costs and carry the risk of life-threatening complications.

Therapeutic Cloning

A promising solution to this remaining problem of histocompatibility would be to create human ES cells genetically identical to the patient. While no ES cells are known to exist in a developed human being and are therefore not available for treatment, such cells could possibly be obtained through the procedure of somatic cell nuclear transfer (NT). In this still largely theoretical procedure, body cells from a patient would be fused with an egg cell that has had its nucleus (including the nuclear DNA) removed. This would theoretically allow the production of a blastocyst-staged embryo genetically identical to the patient that could, in turn, lead to the production of ES cells identical to the patient. In addition, published data suggests that the procedure of NT can "rejuvenate" an aged cell, restoring the proliferative capacity inherent in cells at the beginning of life. Therefore, NT as applied to the production of therapeutic stem cells could have valuable and important applications in the treatment of age-related degenerative diseases.

The use of somatic cell nuclear transfer for the purposes of dedifferentiating a patient's cells for purposes of obtaining undifferentiated stem cells has been designated "Therapeutic Cloning" in the United Kingdom. This terminology is used to differentiate this clinical indication from the use of NT for the cloning of a child which in turn is designated "Reproductive Cloning" in the United Kingdom. In the United Kingdom, the use of NT for therapeutic cloning is being encouraged while legislation has been passed to prohibit reproductive cloning.

Not a Mini-You

Imagine you have Parkinson's disease, which causes the destruction of cells in the brain that make the brain chemical dopamine. Theoretically you could go to Advanced Cell Technology (ACT) [a biotechnology company], provide a skin cell and ask them to make a clone of you. This is called therapeutic cloning because the embryo that is made will never be implanted into a womb and allowed to become a mini-you.

To make the therapeutic clone, scientists fuse the nucleus of your skin cell, which contains your entire DNA, with an egg cell that has had the egg donor's nucleus removed. A few proprietary chemicals are added to trick the egg cell into behaving as if sperm has fertilized it.

If all goes well, the egg cell containing your DNA begins dividing and forms into a blastocyst [four-day old embryo]. The inner cell mass is removed and the stem cells are then converted into dopamine-producing brain cells. Theoretically, these cells will not be rejected by your immune system when implanted into your brain.

Tim Friend, *USA Today*, July 17, 2001.

As promising as NT technologies may be in the arena of therapeutic cloning, a remaining difficulty would be on a source of human oocytes [eggs before maturation], both for research purposes, but also eventually for large-scale clinical implementation. We believe there may be certain advantages to the use of "surrogate" oocytes from animal sources. Animal oocytes could be supplied in large numbers on an economical basis, they could be "humanized" so as to provide fully human cells with human, rather than animal, mitochondria, and they could also potentially be engineered to be defective in producing a fetus even if used in an inappropriate effort to clone a human being by implantation in a uterus. Since these oocytes would be produced in cloned animals (presumably cows), they could, in principle, offer two advantages: 1) an economical and ethically acceptable source of oocytes for therapeutic cloning, and 2) it is possible that they could be engineered to be effective in dedifferentiating human cells and allowing differentiation into specific lineages, but defective in creating a human embryo if implanted into a uterus. This may prevent the abuse of the technology in the event of an inappropriate use of the technology in attempting to produce a pregnancy.

Not for Cloning a Human Being

The NT technologies described above are not designed to be used for the cloning of a human being. Advanced Cell Technology [a major biotechnical company] has no intent to clone a human being, and we are opposed to efforts to clone a human being. As of today, we see no clear utility in producing a child by NT, and even if such uses were identified, NT would likely carry with it an inappropriately high risk of embryonic and fetal wastage. However, we believe that the production of genetically engineered surrogate animal oocytes may be an important resource for medical research, and may solve certain practical and ethical problems associated with sourcing human oocytes and the risks of abuse in human reproductive cloning.

It should be emphasized that the above-mentioned technologies are still in the very earliest stages of development. It is not possible as of today to determine whether the production of human ES cells through sexual or asexual means will meet all the necessary requirements for the development of human therapeutics. What is clear, however, is that a careful, informed, and reasoned public discourse would help insure that these technologies could develop to the point where they could be used in the clinic to treat human disease.

Ethical Considerations

The problem of sourcing human cells and tissues for transplantation raises numerous ethical dilemmas. Because developing embryonic and fetal cells and tissues are "young" and are still in the process of forming mature tissues, there has been considerable interest in obtaining these tissues for use in human medicine. However, the use of aborted embryo or fetal tissue raises numerous issues ranging from concerns over increasing the frequency of elected abortion, to simple issues of maintaining quality controls standards in this hypothetical industry. Similarly, obtaining cells and tissues from living donors or cadavers is also not without ethical issues. For instance, an important and largely unresolved issue is whether it is morally acceptable to keep "deceased" individuals on life support for long periods of time in order to harvest organs as they are needed.

The implementation of ES-based technologies could address some of the ethical problems described above. First, it is important to note that the production of large numbers of human ES cells would not in itself cause these same concerns in accessing human embryonic or fetal tissue, since the resulting cells have the potential to be grown for very long periods of time. Using only a limited number of human embryos not used during in vitro fertilization procedures, biotechnology could theoretically supply the needs of many millions of patients if the problem of histocompatibility could be resolved. Second, in the case of NT procedures, the patient may be at lower risk of complications in transplant rejection. Third, the only human cells used would be from the patient. Theoretically, the need to access tissue from other human beings could be reduced. . . .

The relevant issue is that the biotechnology industry is seeking guidelines for the application of ES and NT technologies in medicine. We believe that these new technologies, if properly applied, could lead to significant medical advances with lifesaving potential. Poorly constructed legislation, designed to prohibit the cloning of a human being, could inadvertently interfere with urgent and ethical applications of the technologies in medicine.

"'Therapeutic' human cloning is an unnecessary evil."

Therapeutic Human Cloning Should Be Banned

Mae-Wan Ho and Joe Cummins

Numerous scientists object to therapeutic cloning—the creation of human embryos for the generation of human tissue for medical treatments. In the following viewpoint, scientists Mae-Wan Ho and Joe Cummins argue that such cloning is morally unacceptable and is a dangerous step toward reproductive cloning and the genetic engineering of humans. The authors argue that adult stem cells, like embryonic stem cells, can be used to create a wide variety of human tissue, making therapeutic human cloning unnecessary. Ho is founder and director of the Institute of Science in Society (I-SIS), a nonprofit organization based in London, England, that seeks to maintain social responsibility within the fields of scientific research and application. Cummins is professor emeritus of genetics at the University of West Ontario in London, Ontario, Canada.

As you read, consider the following questions:
1. According to the authors, what is a blastocyst?
2. How do Ho and Cummins support their claim that the use of embryonic stem cells is risky?
3. In Ho and Cummins's opinion, why is there a great commercial interest in embryonic stem cells?

S tem cells are cells in mammals including human beings that have the ability to divide and give rise to specialized, differentiated cells. The fertilized egg cell possesses this ability to the highest degree, for it has the potential to divide and develop into the entire organism with the full complement of cell types. The fertilized egg cell is *totipotent*.

Totipotency is retained as the egg divides into two and even four cells, so that each cell, when separated, is capable of developing into a complete foetus. That is how twins, triplets and quadruplets come about; they are natural human clones with identical genetic *and* cytoplasmic makeup.

When the embryo is four days old, and after several rounds of cell division, a hollow sphere is formed, called a *blastocyst*, within which is a cluster of cells called the *inner cell mass*. The outer layer is destined to form the placenta and other supporting tissues needed for the development of the foetus in the womb. The inner cell mass will go on to become all the tissues of the foetus' body. These cells are no longer totipotent, but *pluripotent*, ie, they can give rise to many types of cells, but not all of the ones required for foetal development.

As development proceeds, the inner cell mass divides further and becomes more restricted in the range of cells they will become. For example, blood stem cells will eventually give rise to red blood cells, white blood cells and platelets, and skin stem cells will give rise to all the various types of skin cells. These more specialized stem cells are said to be *multipotent*.

Pluripotent and multipotent stem cells in the embryo came to be known as *embryonic stem cells* or ES cells.

Restricted in Use?

Stem cells are also found in children and adults; these are known as *adult stem cells*. Blood stem cells, for example, are found in the bone marrow of every child and adult, and in very small numbers, also in the blood stream; they continually replace the supply of blood cells throughout life. Recently, adult stem cells have also been found in brain as well as muscle, liver, skin and other tissues.

One of the main arguments used in favour of 'therapeutic' human embryo cloning is that adult stem cells are much more restricted in their potential to become different cell types than ES cells. However, it is beginning to appear that adult stem cells have the potential to give rise to a far greater range of cell types than previously imagined, and stunning results have been obtained. Furthermore, there are ways to obtain ES cells other than human cloning.

Not All Equal

There are three kinds of ES cells. The first is derived from the inner cell mass, a procedure pioneered in Dr. James Thomson's laboratory in the University of Wisconsin using 'excess' embryos from *in vitro* fertilization clinics. The second, embryonic germ cells, is isolated from the regions of the embryo destined to become ovaries or testes. This was first carried out by Dr. John Gearhart's group in Johns Hopkins University, using foetuses from terminated pregnancies. The cells resulting from the two laboratories appear to be very similar.

Undiscovered Bounty?

Nobody ever heard of this incredibly important research on human embryos until 10 minutes ago. Yet everyone makes believe he's known about the undiscovered bounty in human embryos forever, and talks about it with real moral indignation. This whole debate is a hoax designed to trick Americans into yielding ground on human experimentation.

Ann Coulter, *Human Events*, July 30, 2001.

The third kind of ES cells involves somatic cell nuclear transfer, the technique that created Dolly, the lamb cloned from a cell of an adult sheep. Researchers take a normal human (or animal) unfertilised egg and remove the nucleus, replacing it with the nucleus from a somatic cell of a human donor. The perceived advantage of this procedure is that the somatic cell donor could be the patient requiring tissue replacement, thus avoiding problems associated with immune rejection of transplanted cells or tissues that are foreign to the body.

As is clear from the description, the first two categories of ES cells do not involve the creation of human embryos, and research on those ES cells has already been going on for years. Many people may find research on those stem cells morally acceptable, though it will be difficult to justify research on those cells in view of the latest discoveries on the enormous developmental potentials of adult cells (see below), which make ES cells completely redundant.

Serious Moral Concerns

It is research on ES cells obtained by nuclear transfer that raises the most serious moral concerns, for it requires the creation of embryos specifically for providing ES cells, the embryos being destroyed in the process.

In December 1998, researchers in the Infertility Clinic at Kyeonghee University in Korea announced that they had successfully cloned a human embryo by transferring the nucleus from the somatic cell of a 30 year old woman into one of her unfertilized eggs. This embryo was reported to have developed to the fourth cell division stage, when it would have been implanted. But it was destroyed on ethical considerations. Meanwhile, researchers in the United States and Australia have created 'human' embryos by transferring the nucleus of human cells into the eggs of a cow and a pig. It is of course questionable whether the embryos created by such procedures are human, and whether they are justifiable on moral grounds. These were destroyed at day 14. It was not clear, however, whether ES cells had been extracted from the embryos before they were destroyed.

Proponents claim that one of the major advantages of ES cells is that established cell lines can be obtained only from ES cells and not adult stem cells; though this may no longer be true (see below).

ES cells carry health risks, and there are major technical difficulties in creating them with nuclear transplant cloning techniques.

- ES cells can give rise to teratomas—malignant tumours (cancers) consisting of a disorganized mass of differentiated cells—on being transplanted.
- Nuclear transplant cloning is a very inefficient process with massive failure rates, requiring a large number of donor eggs.

- Nuclear transplant clones created by transferring human nuclei into cow and pig egg carry even greater risks, as it is well-known that such interspecific nuclear-cytoplasmic hybrids fail to develop normally.

Commercial Interests, Not Public Good

There are powerful commercial interests in ES stem cells. Geron Corporation of Menlo Park, California, gained first rights to exploit cells commercially, and also funded the isolation of embryonic germ cells. A total of ten companies were involved in exploiting stem cell technology and stem cells in 2000. Geron already owns dozens of patents on ES cells.

Companies investing in adult stem cell technology include Nexell Therapeutics of Irvine, California, and Anastrom Biosciences of Ann Arbor. Osiris Therapeutics of Baltimore identified mesenchyme stem in the supportive tissue that surrounds the bone marrow, and has patented systems for isolating and producing those cells, and launched two clinical trials. Mesenchyme cells can differentiate into cartilage, muscle and even neurons. Neural stem cells came on the scene later, but already clinical trials have begun.

It is clear that the major impetus for both ES and adult stem cell research is coming from the biotech companies and scientists working with them. Therapy is likely to be very costly on account of the multiple license fees that have to be paid, not only on cells and cell lines but on isolation procedures.

Public opposition to 'therapeutic' human embryo cloning has been fierce. Apart from the moral objection to the creation of human embryos that are destined to be destroyed, many groups feel that 'therapeutic' human cloning is a slippery slope to reproductive cloning and the re-emergence of eugenics. The Clinton administration had forbidden such research in federally funded projects; and no European Government, with the exception of the United Kingdom, is in favour of such research. . . .

Promises of Adult Stem Cells

Mammals appear to contain some 20 major types of somatic stem cells. Stem cells have been described that can generate all the cells in the brain, the liver, pancreas, bone and cartilage.

These adult stem cells are increasingly found to have the potential to become practically as many different cell types as ES cells. Furthermore, it appears that differentiated adult cells can be made to revert to cells remarkably similar to stem cells, and to have the ability to multiply for long periods in cell culture. Some of the findings are highlighted below.

• Mouse bone marrow stem cells can give rise to skeletal muscle and brain cells. Liver/pancreas stem cells can give rise to blood cells and brain cells. Brain cells can give rise to all previous cell types including the peripheral nervous system and smooth muscle. Brain cells have been found to differentiate to muscle, blood, intestine, liver and heart.

• Catherine Verfaillie of the University of Minnesota in Minneapolis is reported to have isolated bone marrow cells from children and adults that can become brain, liver, and muscle cells as well. These were found in adults between 45 and 50 years old. This research has not yet appeared in print.

• Scientists from the National Neurological Institute and Stem Cell Research Institute in Milan, Italy, succeeded in growing skeletal muscle from stem cells originating from an adult brain, both in culture and in animals receiving the transplanted stem cells.

• A researcher in Britain, Dr. Ilham Abuljadaye, has just announced an efficient method for creating large quantities of adult stem cells from white blood cells, and her findings have been independently replicated, though not yet published. The method involves inducing the white blood cells to de-differentiate in the test-tube into stem cells. That means it will be feasible to prepare stem cells from the patient who is in need of cell or tissue transplant, greatly simplifying the procedure, avoiding immune reactions and reducing cost.

• Two research teams at University College London found that adult rat cells can be made to divide hundreds of times when provided with the right mixture of nutrients, and without taking on the undesirable characteristics of cancer cells, such as uncontrollable growth. Adult human cells may have the same capacity.

• Another possibility is that the patient's own stem cells could be stimulated to multiply and replace cells and tissues within the body itself.

We reject research on ES cells created by human 'therapeutic' cloning on the following grounds.

- It is totally unnecessary, given the promise of adult stem cells and adult cells from the patients themselves, which can be most effectively used for cell and tissue replacement.
- It is morally unacceptable to create human embryos for providing ES cells.
- It is a slippery slope to human reproductive cloning.
- Nuclear transplant cloning has very low success rates and generates many abnormalities.
- Cloning procedures involving transplanting human nuclei into animal eggs carry even greater risks.
- ES cells are already available using 'excess' embryos from *in vitro* fertilization clinics and aborted foetuses.
- ES cells carry cancer risks on being transplanted.
- ES cells are subject to multiple patents, on cloning and isolation procedures as well as on the cells themselves; this will make their use in cell or tissue replacement therapy very costly.
- Adult stem cells are already showing great promise in cell and tissue replacement and are likely to be much less costly.

'Therapeutic' human cloning is an unnecessary evil.

Periodical Bibliography

The following articles have been selected to supplement the diverse views presented in this chapter. Addresses are provided for periodicals not indexed in the *Readers' Guide to Periodical Literature*, the *Alternative Press Index*, the *Social Sciences Index*, or the *Index to Legal Periodicals and Books*.

Jonathan R. Cohen	"In God's Garden," *Hastings Center Report*, July 1999.
Jonathan Colvin	"Me, My Clone, and I (or in Defense of Human Cloning)," *Humanist*, May 2000.
Dinesh D'Souza	"Technopia or Techno-Hell," *American Enterprise*, December 2000.
Ronald M. Green	"Should We Be Working Toward Human Cloning for Infertility Treatment?" *Contemporary OB/GYN*, May 2000.
Neil Munro and Marilyn Werber Serafini	"Now a Debate, in Triplicate, over Cloning," *National Journal*, April 14, 2001.
Nation	"Send in the Clones . . ." October 8, 2001.
Barry A. Palevitz	"Stem Cells and Cloning in the Public Eye," *Scientist*, September 3, 2001.
Jonathan Rauch	"Sure, You Can Clone Mozart, but You Can't Reproduce Him," *Los Angeles Times*, August 20, 2001.
Thomas Shannon	"The Rush to Clone: It Is Unethical to Apply This Unproven Research to Humans," *America*, September 10, 2001.
Gunjan Sinha	"A Clone of Our Own," *Popular Science*, January 2000.
Abraham Verghese	"Cell Block: Proposed Limits on Stem-Cell Research and Bans on Cloning Cut Off Something Else Too: Hope," *New York Times Magazine*, August 19, 2001.
Wall Street Journal	"The House Was Right to Ban Cloning," August 2, 2001.
Washington Post	"Reasons Not to Clone," April 1, 2001.
Sondra Wheeler	"Making Babies?" *Sojourners*, May 1999.
Ian Wilmut	"Breaking the Clone Barrier," *Time*, March 29, 1999.

CHAPTER 2

What Ethics Should Guide Organ Donations?

Chapter Preface

A new definition of death has been established to include permanently comatose or vegetative patients who depend on life-support machines to stay alive. This redefinition of death is critical to the procurement of organs for donation because it has greatly expanded the pool of organ donors.

Comatose or vegetative patients are routinely sought after as organ donors when families and doctors decide to "pull the plug" because their organs are largely intact and functional. In these cases, doctors perceive death as the permanent absence of neurological activity, or "brain death." A Harvard Medical School committee conceptualized brain death in a 1968 publication. However, brain death did not become a legal term until the Uniform Definition of Death Act was drafted in 1980. It describes death as being "the irreversible cessation of all functions of the entire brain, including the brain stem," or "whole-brain death." Proponents of whole-brain death suggest that it is useful because it humanely allows patients to be removed from life support and increases the number of organs available for transplantation.

However, critics believe that the concept of whole-brain death should be challenged because it is ambiguous. On one side, some commentators claim that whole-brain death is too wide a definition and leaves too many vegetative and comatose patients on life support when there is no hope for recovery. According to medical ethicist R.M. Veatch, one is dead when there is "higher-brain death," the irreversible loss of cognitive function, although primitive neurological functions may be intact. On the contrary, others reject all concepts of brain death. For instance, Robert D. Truog, a professor of anesthesia, maintains that tests used to analyze neurological activity are flawed, rendering living, breathing, thinking patients vulnerable to euthanasia and organ harvesting.

In the following chapter, authors discuss whether or not efforts used to ameliorate the organ shortage, such as the establishment of brain death, are ethically sound.

"*We should learn to transcend the strong, visceral opposition to organ sales that functions as the emotional anchor to present policy.*"

The Sale of Organs for Transplants Should Be Legalized

Richard A. Epstein

Richard A. Epstein is the James Parker Hall Distinguished Service Professor of Law at the University of Chicago and author of *Mortal Peril: Our Inalienable Right to Health Care?* In the following viewpoint, Epstein asserts that selling organs for transplants should be allowed because relying on altruism for organ procurement has resulted in a shortage of organs. He insists that a system of voluntary exchange, whether the donor is rewarded with money or other types of compensation, will increase the supply of organs for transplants.

As you read, consider the following questions:

1. According to Epstein, what are the fundamentals of voluntary exchange?
2. How does the author counter the view that organ sales should remain banned because patients are unable to make rational decisions about risky procedures?
3. How does Epstein respond to the argument that a free market of organs will exploit the poor?

In the United States, it is honorable to donate one's organs but illegal to sell them.

It is easy to praise those who donate organs to others. Live donations—such as a mother giving a son a kidney— require tremendous sacrifice that only a donor's love and fortitude can overcome. Donations made at the time of death—called cadaveric donations—require family members to aid a perfect stranger in their unexpected moment of grief. It's hard not to laud such selflessness.

But in lauding donations, why condemn sales? Although the culture holds that buying and selling of organs is highly distasteful, a good argument for such sales is beginning to be made, albeit tentatively, in this country.

Indeed, we should learn to transcend the strong, visceral opposition to organ sales that functions as the emotional anchor to present policy. Too long have we relied in vain on the drumbeat for altruism to reduce the dreadful shortage of available organs.

Considerable Social Cost

To consider the argument for organ sales, start with the fundamentals of voluntary exchange. The affection we have for family and intimate friends does not carry over to the vast world of strangers. Yet, as self-interested strangers, we need to cooperate to survive, and the contract of sale, like other forms of voluntary exchange, is one way to do that. Each of us exchanges something he values for something he values more. The repeated process of exchange increases the supply of desired goods and directs them to the individuals who value them most.

Look at it this way: A mother might well give her kidney to her son; indeed about 25 percent of kidney donations are live donations. But asked to donate to a stranger, she would probably recoil at the obvious costs: loss of a kidney, the pain of surgery, the long recovery, some diminished physical capacity, and some risk of death. Yet the need by that stranger is just as real. And too often in this country such needs are going unmet—at considerable social cost.

Put simply, a world in which 100 individuals each have one kidney is a world with higher expected benefits than a world in which 50 people each have two kidneys and the other 50, with failing kidneys, face dialysis or death. And even if we allow for some failure and slippage, the anticipated gains still remain positive.

Cash (or indeed any other form of compensation, such as insurance) might be the engine to move us to the preferred outcome of more lives saved. No one can be sure that a voluntary market will emerge just because it is allowed. Even so, nothing justifies the moral denunciations hurled at those of us who look to sales to unlock these potential social gains.

Note the alternative: As surgeons become more skilled and the numbers of sudden, traumatic deaths continue their welcome decline, the shortage in available organs increases inexorably. For kidneys we have seen the waiting lists continue their relentless expansion from about 13,000 in 1988 to nearly 40,000 in 1998. Parallel increases are found for other organs.

Verging on Irrationality?

So why not legalize the sale of organs, whether from live or dead individuals, in the hopes of expanding supply? The dogged defenders of the status quo throw up arguments against any form of social experiment. We are told, for example, that organ sales must be banned because individuals verge on irrationality, unable to make informed judgments about the risks they assume.

But complex surgery also tests rational decision making, and we do not ban experimental treatments because some patients are easily confused. Nor do we ban live organ donations even though families may put enormous pressure on one of their own to make an uncompensated transfer. Rather, we supply potential donors information in the first case and donors independent advice in the second. Confusion and pressure in combination rarely justify banning a practice with lifesaving potential.

We can invest a bit more in legal infrastructure to preserve most of the benefits of voluntary exchange while largely curbing transactions tainted by mistake or coercion.

Defenders of the current ban also claim that it prevents unfair exploitation of the most vulnerable segments of our population, those who are desperate enough to sell their organs for cash. But the poor and the disadvantaged will not be sought after, let alone exploited, because they do not make ideal candidates for organ transfers. Quite the opposite.

The risk of alcoholism, hepatitis, or AIDS is every bit as dangerous with organ donations as with blood donations. Organized markets would keep these people out of the system by concentrating on that smaller sliver of the population in excellent health but which has some powerful financial reason to take the quite extreme step of selling organs: a child's operation, for example, or a relative trapped in horrible circumstances overseas.

Financial Incentives

Although altruism can be a powerful factor in motivating organ donations, it works best within families and cannot be expected to function as efficiently in the market for cadaveric organs. Individuals may sign anatomical donor cards indicating their wishes, but in practice, procurement agencies will remove organs only with familial consent. Thus, to increase supply, it is necessary to provide families with additional incentives. This is especially true given the relatively few deaths (10,000 to 12,000 annually) that occur in such a way that the deceased's organs are suitable for transplantation.

To increase donations, we need to consider financial incentives mimicking those that prices provide in a market economy. Perhaps the simplest approach is to give tax incentives to families who agree to donate.

Charles T. Carlstrom and Christy D. Rollow, *Cato Journal*, Fall 1997.

Most potential sellers would decline to offer an organ for sale, even if it were legal, but so what? Universal participation isn't needed to erase the shortfall in available, lifesaving organs; only a tiny fraction of the population need participate to do that.

Still, a well-functioning market might be quickly filled. Its volume of business would allow the emergence of stable prices and sensible procurement procedures. If there were bumps along the way, it would not be for the first time.

Right now, even with organ donations, the process is frequently stymied because of uncertainty over who controls disposition of the organs of a deceased person. By law, families and transplant teams should be allowed to honor organ donation cards. But in practice virtually every close family member is given a veto over the donation process. Allowing the donation cards (at least when recently reaffirmed) to control the decision could expedite both gifts and sales, with the payment, if any, going as the organ donor directs, or failing that, to the next of kin.

Critics argue further that any sales of organs will drive out voluntary donations, and do nothing to alleviate the present shortage. But it is unlikely that the substitution of sales for gifts would be at a one-to-one level. It is unlikely that all donors would want cash, but even if they did, the dangers of organ sales to the procurement process are hard to detect.

Right now organs are, in a fashion, sold anyway. Concealed from public view, transplant centers wage fierce competition for cadaveric organs to pave the way for the sale of transplantation services from $100,000 and up. But it is doctors and transplant centers that implicitly capture the proceeds from sale.

Allowing individuals to sell organs need not increase the total bill to organ recipients. Instead it will redirect some portion of the gain to the party who transfers the organ.

At the same time, the change in legal regime should change the price of transplant surgery, and cut down on the amount of wasteful jockeying that takes place for desired organs. We have no shortage of transplant teams, only a shortage of organs. The sensible national policy should be directed to eliminating that blockage in the system.

A Crabbed Set of Assumptions

Finally, it will be said that a sales policy will favor the rich over the poor in the procurement of organs. But the rich are already favored, if only because of their willingness to go anywhere instantly for treatment. At worse, that inequity continues in an open market, as the rich are more able to afford organs than the poor. But nothing prevents the government from using tax dollars to purchase organs for the needy poor.

In short, the concern with the distribution of benefits should not be allowed to thwart the increase in the number of persons benefited.

Taken as a whole, the current policy rests on a crabbed set of assumptions that underestimates the intelligence and rationality of ordinary people. Their constant negativism prevents experimentation with the one set of social practices known to reduce shortages elsewhere, and thus prevents us from acquiring the information that allows for sensible modification and regulation of the system.

We need to get past our own squeamishness and give those who need it another chance to live.

| "*Our society has very strong reasons not to allow the transfer of organs from the living or the dead for money.*"

The Sale of Organs for Transplants Should Not Be Legalized

James F. Childress

In the following viewpoint, James F. Childress argues that permitting the sale and purchase of human organs presents serious social risks. Placing a market value on human organs is likely to commodify the human body, he contends. In addition, creating a market in organ procurement places poor and disadvantaged people at risk for coercion and exploitation. Childress is director of the Institute for Practical Ethics at the University of Virginia and coauthor of *Principles of Biomedical Ethics.*

As you read, consider the following questions:
1. How does the author support his view that allowing organs to be sold would not increase their supply?
2. According to Childress, how can the system of organ donation be improved?
3. How does Childress respond to the proposal to offer financial incentives or rewards for organ donation?

Excerpted from "Q: Should Congress Allow the Buying and Selling of Human Organs? No," by James F. Childress, *Insight*, May 7, 2001. Reprinted with permission.

The number of patients awaiting an organ transplant exceeded 75,000 in late March 2001. Yet in 1999, the last year for which there are complete figures, there only were 21,655 transplants with organs from 4,717 living donors and 5,859 from cadavers (many of which provided more than one organ). Organ donation continues to fall further and further behind the demand for organs, and new initiatives have failed to reduce the gap. In this situation, why shouldn't we turn to the free market to increase the supply of transplantable organs, which can save lives and improve the quality of life?

From a System of Gifts

Buying or selling an organ isn't always morally wrong. We don't, and shouldn't, always condemn those who sell or purchase an organ. We can understand why someone might do so. But should we change our laws to permit sales of organs and even enforce contracts to sell organs? Should we turn away from a system of gifts to a market in organs?

Our society has very strong reasons not to allow the transfer of organs from the living or the dead for money. In presenting these reasons, it is useful to separate the acquisition of organs from their distribution. Normally, acquisition and distribution go together. However, if those who need organs had to purchase them directly, then the poor would end up selling organs to the rich—a distribution that would strike many as unfair. Thus, let's assume that the government or a private organization under government regulation will purchase organs and then distribute them in a fair and equitable way. I'll call this an "organ-procurement market."

Such a market could target living donors or cadaveric sources of organs. I use the term "sources" because those who sell their organs are not donors, they are sellers or vendors. Let's begin with cadaveric organs removed after an individual's death.

The main argument for rescinding the federal prohibition on the sale of organs is based on utility—allowing the sale of organs would increase their supply. But would a market actually increase the number of cadaveric organs for transplantation? Despite the claims of market fundamentalists, we simply do not know whether a market would reduce the scarcity of organs, in contrast to many other goods. And we have good reasons to be skeptical.

An Unnecessary Route

Indeed, I will argue, we shouldn't legalize a market in organ procurement because it probably would be ineffective, perhaps counterproductive (in reducing donations and possibly even the overall number of organs available for transplantation) and likely change our attitudes and practices by commodifying the human body and its parts. Furthermore, it is unnecessary to take this route, with all its problems, because we can make the system of donation effective without such ethical risks.

It would be unwise to move away from a system of donation unless we have good evidence that a market actually would increase the supply of organs. After all, organ donations provide a substantial (though insufficient) number of organs. Some evidence against a potential market's effectiveness in cadaveric organ procurement comes from the reasons people now give for not signing donor cards. One proponent of the market contends that people now fail to donate "because of inertia, mild doubts about their preferences, a slight distaste for considering the subject or the inconvenience involved in completing or carrying a donor card." If these reasons for nondonation were the only ones, a market in cadaveric organ procurement probably would work. In fact, however, opinion polls indicate that fears of being declared dead prematurely or having one's death hastened in order to provide organs seriously inhibit many from signing donor cards.

The fears and distrust that limit organ donation would render utterly ineffective a system of organ procurement based on sales. A futures market—whereby individuals contract now for delivery of organs upon their deaths—is the most defensible because people sell their own, not others', organs. However, if people at present are reluctant to sign donor cards because they fear they may not receive proper care in the hospital, imagine their fears about accepting money for the delivery of usable organs upon their deaths.

Once they have signed the contract, all that remains for its fulfillment is their death. And a regulated market would not eliminate their fears. After all, such fears persist in our regulated system of organ donation.

Turning Bodies into Commodities

Critics often contend that allowing sales of organs would turn bodies and parts into commodities. Such commodification could lead us to think about and treat dead bodies in merely instrumental terms, thereby damaging important social values. In addition, many claim, commodification could damage and even reduce altruism. A market in organs would drive out, or very substantially reduce, organ donations, in part because it would redefine acts of donating organs. No longer would donors provide the "gift of life"—they instead would donate the equivalent of the market value of the organs provided.

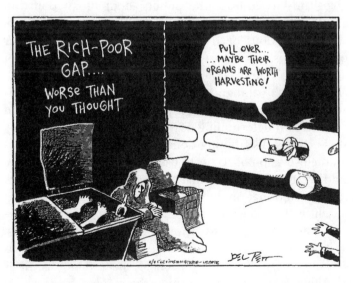

Pett. © 1995 by *Lexington Herald-Leader*. Reprinted by permission of the author.

In short, market defenders have not proposed an effective system to obtain additional cadaveric organs. Not only would a procurement market probably be ineffective, it could be counterproductive and have other social costs. Its financial costs would not be negligible. Furthermore, the system of donation has features, including its connection with altruism, that make it ethically preferable, other things being equal. And we can make our system of express donation more effective.

It works fairly well now. For example, according to some estimates, the acts of cadaveric-organ donation in 1999 represented close to half of the patients who died in circumstances where their organs could be salvaged for transplantation (usually following brain death). It might be possible, and desirable, to expand the categories of potential donors to include many who die according to cardiopulmonary standards. Beyond expanding the criteria of donor eligibility, we need to work to make effective the recently adopted policy of required referral. This policy mandates referral to an organ-procurement organization that can then ask the family about organ donation.

Programs to educate the public about organ donation must attend to attitudes of distrust and mistrust, not merely to the tremendous need for organs. It is difficult to alter those attitudes, but increasing the public's understanding of brain death certainly is one way to proceed.

The public's willingness to donate cadaveric organs generally presupposes trust not only in the society's criteria and procedures for determining death, but in its criteria for fairly and effectively distributing donated organs as well. In addition, the provision of access to basic health care for everyone would create a sense of solidarity that dramatically could increase organ donation, but that vision is a distant one.

I salute the decisions in some states to give the decedent's signed donor card priority over family objections, but it is even more important to educate individuals as members of families. They need to share their decisions with their families and consider their roles as potential donors of a family member's organs. Donor cards may be a useful mechanism to stimulate such conversations, but in and of themselves they are too individualistic, legalistic and formalistic. The process of intrafamilial communication is more important.

Recognizing and Honoring Donors

Society also provides various incentives for organ donation, such as by recognizing and honoring donors in various ways. Would it be possible to offer some financial incentives without crossing over into a market for organ procurement? Consider the following: As a regular expression of its gratitude for organ donation, society could cover the decedent's funeral expenses up to a certain amount, perhaps $1,000 or more. In this way, the community would recognize with gratitude the decedent's and/or the family's act of donation and also pay respects to the donor or source of the organs by sharing in the disposition of his/her final remains.

Any proposal for such "rewarded gifting" will require careful scrutiny, in part because organ donation is such a highly sensitive area, marked by complex beliefs, symbols, attitudes, sentiments and practices, some of them religious in nature. But a carefully conceived pilot experiment, such as providing death benefits—as Pennsylvania has discussed—may be justifiable. However, it may infringe current laws. In any event, it requires the utmost caution because of its risks. One risk is that it will be perceived as purchasing organs rather than as expressing gratitude and providing incentives for donation.

Coercion and Exploitation

I have focused on cadaveric organs, but what about a market in organ procurement from living individuals? Such a market probably would be more effective than a futures market in cadaveric organs—more individuals probably would be willing to part with a kidney, especially with reduced risks from kidney removal and with generous compensation. However, the social risk of commodification—of treating living human bodies and their parts as commodities—is very troubling. In addition, the risks of coercion and exploitation, especially of poor people, are substantial. The assertion of a moral right to sell a kidney against the legal prohibition of such a sale is not persuasive; we have good reasons, based on concerns about commodification, coercion and exploitation, to reject such sales as incompatible with our moral vision of the kind of society to which we aspire.

Vigorous efforts along the paths I have indicated should obviate the need to adopt a market in organ procurement, whether from living or cadaveric sources. We have little reason to believe that a futures market will be effective in obtaining cadaveric organs and considerable reason to worry about the risks and social costs of such a market, as well as a market for living organ procurement. We should just say "no" to both markets.

"*Unless there is a majority view against change, the contracting out [presumed consent] system of organ donation should be introduced.*"

Presumed Consent for Organ Donation Is Ethical

I. Kennedy, R.A. Sells, A.S. Daar, R.D. Guttmann, R. Hoffenberg, M. Lock, J. Radcliffe-Richards, and N. Tilney

A system of presumed consent for organ procurement defines every person as an organ donor unless they clearly indicate that they do not wish to donate their organs during their lifetime. In the following viewpoint, the authors support a policy of presumed consent in order to relieve the organ shortage. They claim that countries practicing presumed consent have significantly increased their supply of organs in an ethical manner. The authors are members of the International Forum for Transplant Ethics, a nonprofit worldwide organization aimed at increasing the public's awareness of the importance and need for organ donations.

As you read, consider the following questions:
1. According to the authors, in Italy, when can organs be removed from a body when the individual does not consent to it during life?
2. In the authors' opinion, for what reasons do organ donations vary from country to country?
3. How do the authors define the property claims of a deceased person's relatives?

Is there a moral case for changing the law regulating organ donation from a system of "contracting in" to "contracting out" or "presumed consent" in those countries that have not yet done so? Contracting in refers to a system in which the law requires that donors and/or relatives must positively indicate their willingness for organs to be removed for transplantation. In a contracting out system, organs may be removed after death unless individuals positively indicate during their lifetimes that they did not wish this to be done, a system also known as presumed consent.

We start with the premise that any measure that increases the supply of organs for transplantation is a good thing. If the contracting out system were to achieve this, the onus would then be on those who oppose it to demonstrate that the benefit that flows from it is outweighed by the harm.

Since 1990 in those countries that have a contracting in system in place the number of cadaver organs available for transplantation has not kept up with demand; indeed the gap is widening. Nonetheless, many people believe that the law should not be changed, arguing that a significant improvement in supply could result from public and professional education and measures to simplify the process of donation and retrieval of organs. Although not discounting this possibility, we believe that a contracting out system would achieve the same effect with greater certainty, as has been shown in countries that have changed to this option. Therefore we believe that it is morally unjustified to perpetuate a system that falls short of increasing the availability of organs to people who might benefit from transplantation.

Current Situation

The guiding principles issued by the World Health Organization (WHO) in 1991 state that organs may be removed from the body of a dead person if: (a) any consents required by law are obtained; and (b) there is no reason to believe that in the absence of any formal consent given during life the dead person would have objected to such removal.

In countries where transplantation is widely practised, the law permits removal of organs from the cadaver of a person who made known the wish to donate while alive. In practice most people have not made any such formal declaration. In these circumstances the law looks to the relatives for consent. Since most donors will have spent some time in the intensive care unit before death is pronounced, the relatives will be present when the decision is taken to withdraw life support and are then approached. They decide whether organs may be removed and used for transplantation, and their power is in turn laid down by the law.

Far-Reaching Benefits

Ideally, if a presumed consent policy could be effectively implemented and well monitored, the benefits could be quite far-reaching. It is estimated that there are at least 11,000 cadaveric donors potentially available each year; yet, because consent is often not attainable (either due to refusal or failure to locate the family), only about 4500 donors are actually obtained. If donation was the standard procedure, there would be a much larger pool of donors, which not only means that greater numbers of people on waiting lists could be given transplants, but that there might be greater chances for tissue matches with patients from among the pool, and in the end, less chance of rejection.

Michelle Wong, *Richmond Journal of Law and Public Interest*, 1998.

The laws of different countries fall into five categories. In the absence of a wish expressed by the donor during life, organs may be removed in the following circumstances.

- Only with the consent of the person lawfully in possession of the body and subject to express objection of the deceased or objection of the relatives, if available (UK).
- After the relatives have been informed of the intention to remove organs, but irrespective of their consent (except for that of the nearest relative, Norway).
- Once it has been ascertained that the relatives do not object (Italy).
- Where the dead person had not expressed an objection, this is confirmed by the relatives and consent is then presumed (Belgium).
- Irrespective of the relatives' views (Austria).

The difference in the rates of organ donation between

countries can be explained by several factors, such as the supply of potential donors (which may vary according to the rate of road-traffic accidents or gun laws, for example), religious and cultural responses to death and to the body after death, and practical issues—eg, the number of intensive-care beds available. Adverse publicity can seriously reduce the supply by reducing the number of potential donors or the consent of relatives. Supply can be increased by energetic educational campaigns, by having more transplant coordinators, by the provision of specialist teams to take over the care of potential donors, and by provision of financial incentives to encourage doctors and institutions to refer patients. All these factors are independent of the nature of the prevailing law.

In three western countries there is evidence that changing to a contracting out system resulted in an increase in organs—Spain, Austria, and Belgium—but the change in legislation has not achieved this rise on its own. In Spain, for example, additional measures included the appointment of more co-ordinators and provision of financial incentives. In the case of Belgium there is well-documented and convincing evidence that a change in the law from contracting in to contracting out in 1986 led to an increase in organ supply. Staff at the organ-transplantation centre in Antwerp were strongly opposed to the new law and retained a contracting in policy accompanied by enhanced public and professional education; by contrast, at Leuven the new law was adopted. In Antwerp, organ donation rates remained unchanged; in Leuven they rose from 15 to 40 donors per year over a 3-year period. In the whole country organ donation rose by 55% within 5 years despite a concurrent decrease in the number of organs available from road-traffic accidents. Citizens who wish to opt out of the scheme may register their objection at any Town Hall; since 1986 less than 2% of the population have done so. Use of a computerised register has simplified ascertaining the existence of any objection. In Belgium, despite the existence of this law, doctors are encouraged to approach the relatives in all cases and practitioners may decide against removing the organs if in their opinion this would cause undue distress or for any other valid reason. Less than 10% of families do object compared with 20-30% elsewhere in Europe. Another benefit has been an increase in the number of referrals of cadaver donors from collaborating centres, suggesting that the intensivists have found the new law favourable to donation. It would seem from the Belgian experience that relatives may be reluctant to take a personal decision about the removal of organs, but they find it easier to agree if they are simply confirming the intention of the dead person. If this is so, a contracting out system has a moral benefit of relieving grieving relatives of the burden of deciding about donation at a time of great psychological stress.

A change in the law thus achieves the dual effect of increasing the supply of organs and lessening the distress of relatives. Those who have moral objections to it must produce convincing evidence that the harm that would follow such a change would outweigh these clear benefits.

Possible Moral Objections

The right of the individual to refuse to donate organs.

This right is allowed for both in principle and in practice by the Belgian model, in which objection can be registered by law and doctors have the discretion to desist if they feel that removal of organs will better reflect the individual's wishes to avoid undue distress to the relatives. It is essential to ensure that simple mechanisms for registering an objection are easily available. In developed countries it should not be difficult to ensure that an opportunity is provided whenever any official business is transacted—eg, when applying for a passport or driving licence. The safety mechanism of checking the decision with the relatives should minimise the possibility of erroneous interpretation of the dead person's wishes. We conclude that a sensitive, secure, and robust system could be introduced, preceded by a reasonable period of notice and publicity to give time to those who wish to register their objection. Whether this approach recommends itself to developing countries, where other priorities compete, is a separate matter.

The rights of relatives.

In most legal systems, relatives have no property claim over the body of the deceased. Furthermore, any claim they may seek to assert seems rather weak when set against the claims of the person in need of a transplant. This is not to argue that relatives' interests should be ignored, and indeed the Belgian model takes them into account. This version of the contracting out system, as opposed to one in which the wishes of the relatives are ignored, is consistent with the recommendations of the Conference of European Health Ministers and WHO. The primary role of relatives is thus to corroborate that the dead person did not actually register an objection. They are not put into the position of having to make the decision themselves, but simply to confirm the facts. As a result the refusal rate is much lower.

Possible Counterproductive Consequences

It may be argued that this change in public policy would invoke such social unease and disquiet that people would turn away from the whole concept of transplantation. This has not been the experience in countries that have changed, where, if anything, the general population and medical professionals are happier with the new law than with the old. In Belgium and Spain an increase in organ supply has been achieved despite a fall in the number of potential donors.

Another objection is that the state already has a big enough stake in our lives—eg, through the tax law, and further incursion into our affairs by assuming possession of our body parts and the right to distribute them to others by law would be a step too far. A study by the King's Fund Institute in 1994 concluded that, in the UK, the medical professions, the transplantation community, and the public were split over the ethics of the contracting out law and it would be inappropriate to recommend a change in the law because this might provoke an acrimonious debate that could damage confidence in transplantation technology as a whole. Others may argue that people would feel pressure not to contract out because this would be socially unacceptable. Both arguments are rebutted by the ready acceptance of the law in Belgium and elsewhere, and the immediate benefit it achieved in increasing the supply of organs.

Clearly, from a moral standpoint, the social context in which any law is to operate and any medical action that arises from it must be a significant consideration in determining policy. Before any such law is promulgated, there will have to be an informed public debate and a clear demonstration that it would be morally acceptable to most people. Much of the objection to change would be mitigated by appropriate public education.

We feel that this debate should now take place and, unless there is a majority view against change, the contracting out system of organ donation should be introduced.

*"Presumed consent implies that the state has
first call on our bodies."*

Presumed Consent for Organ Donation Is Unethical

Melanie Phillips

In a system of presumed consent for organ donation, an individual is assumed to be an organ donor unless he or she of-
ficially opts out of organ donation. In the following viewpoint, Melanie Phillips argues that presumed consent
violates an individual's right to his or her body by handing
over ownership to the government. She concludes that the
policy opens the door to abuse and exploitation in medical
practices. Phillips is a writer and columnist for the *Sunday
Times (London)*.

As you read, consider the following questions:
1. According to Phillips, how has the utilitarian viewpoint
   shaped medical practices?
2. How does the author support her claim that refusing to
   donate organs will be perceived as "antisocial"?
3. In Phillips's view, how can presumed consent threaten
   living donors?

The great social philosopher Richard Titmuss wrote in 1970 that when people donated blood they were performing a very particular social duty. In his classic book *The Gift Relationship*, he observed that at the core of the blood transfusion service lay the principle of the "universal stranger". He meant that, since donors didn't know who would be getting their blood, they couldn't prevent anyone they disliked from receiving it. So everyone was treated equally as needy.

It is in this context that the row over the racist kidney donors needs to be set. The Northern General hospital in Sheffield [England] apparently accepted donor kidneys on condition that they were to be transplanted only into white people. It was subsequently revealed that Muslims and other groups had tried elsewhere to lay down similarly restrictive conditions for the use of relatives' organs.

Like giving blood, however, organ donation is an act of altruism that signals we are all part of one human community. The impulse behind both acts is the same one that causes us to stop in the street and tend a dying person. Laying down who can or cannot receive a kidney or a pint of blood is tantamount to refusing to help an injured or dying person because he happens to be black, Jewish or homosexual.

Moral Blackmail

Such an attitude is intolerable and utterly inimical to the principles of the health service. Yet hospitals presented with this situation face a dilemma, because refusing a donor organ means that someone is likely to die. This is just a sharp variant of the institutionalised moral blackmail intrinsic to organ transplants. Unlike blood donation—an undiluted social good—organ transplantation raises acute ethical problems that have been swept under the carpet. Even worse, doctors' leaders are now using this moral blackmail to bully the population.

The British Medical Association (BMA) proposed in July 1999 that, to bump up the number of donated organs, everyone should be assumed to be a donor unless they opted out. This is almost the position taken by John Harris, the bioethics professor, who said earlier in 1999 not only that there should be presumed consent but also that anyone who opted out should have to give a reason. [Presumed consent is currently not mandated in Great Britain.]

The BMA said at the time that Harris was too extreme. Yet here it is, shoulder to shoulder on this coercive and utterly unacceptable abuse of human rights. What about people who forget to opt out or are too ignorant or handicapped to understand? As some doctors have suggested, this will open up the prospect of "stolen" organs being used. It's up to doctors to make their case for organs to be given, not for people to be expected to do so.

A Niggling Requirement

Presumed Consent would do away with that niggling requirement that one designate oneself as willing to be an organ donor. It eradicates that trifling nuisance of having to deal with grieving family members in order to gain permission to gather up the dying person's organs.

It is, by federal law, a *fait accompli*. Each person standing in line at the supermarket or riding the bus with you is simply an organ donor whose heart may beat for him today, and for another tomorrow.

There [is] an option.

Individuals can formally "opt-out," thereby becoming part of a national database.

You arrive in the emergency room, they determine that you are *as good as dead* and ripe for the harvest, but first they check a database to see if you are one of those "ignorant," "uneducated," "superstitious" fools who has elected to covet his own organs.

Cathy Ramey, *Life Advocate*, September/October 1999.

That expectation, though, gets to the nub of this invidious business. Presumed consent implies that the state has first call on our bodies. That is objectionable. It further implies that our bodies have no value, being merely sacks of spare parts. This grotesque utilitarian viewpoint has become the orthodoxy in our medical and legal establishments. It has given rise to the techno-cannibalism of experimentation on embryos or the proposals to clone embryos for "therapeutic" purposes (kicked into touch by the government for the time being).

Individuals have thus become dispensable, in the supposed interest of relieving suffering. It therefore follows that it is actually our duty to offer bits of ourselves to save another's life. Refusing consent becomes accordingly a profoundly antisocial act. Indeed, how can we not be expected to give reasons if we are causing someone else's death by choosing to be buried with our hearts and livers? You think your body belongs to you? Sentimental claptrap! Out with your kidneys immediately!

Utilitarianism Becomes Tyranny

So utilitarianism becomes tyranny. This contempt for the dead slips seamlessly into contempt for the living. If someone is unconscious, why not assume they're dead, since someone else's more useful life might be saved as a result? Indeed, why not ensure they become dead?

Both these things are now happening. Donors are not necessarily dead when their organs are removed. Brainstem death, the definition used to trigger organ removal, does not mean the whole brain has died. Tests for brainstem death leave most of the brain untested. Further tests might well reveal activity in the higher brain. Indeed, so undead are these donors that they often have to be paralysed by drugs since they continue to react to stimulus. Yet they are opened up and their organs removed.

Even more awful prospects are now looming. The courts are allowing doctors to remove feeding and hydration tubes in order to kill patients who are alive but in a persistent vegetative state (PVS). Artificial feeding is said to be "treatment" and can therefore be withdrawn.

If feeding is treatment, though, what is the disease? Like "brainstem death", this is a definition that owes everything to expediency and nothing to the truth. The distress of these patients' relatives deserves unlimited compassion. Nevertheless, some PVS "hopeless" cases have recovered consciousness; and even where they do not, allowing doctors to kill them is a Rubicon [boundary] that should never have been crossed.

Now the BMA wants to go even further. It says doctors should be able to withdraw feeding and hydration without even going to court, and it would apply this not just to PVS or stroke patients but even to people suffering mental illness who can't give their informed consent. So because human life is deemed to have no intrinsic value, certain human lives are now valueless on criteria to be decided by medical experts. We become expendable.

No More than the Sum of Its Parts

Put together these various developments and you get the prospect of PVS patients being starved to death so that their organs can be used for transplant. This is not some melodramatic fantasy. In 1995 the Law Commission's report on mental incapacity laid out legal criteria to permit the withdrawal of artificial nutrition and hydration from patients who couldn't give their consent. It also said medical or surgical procedures could be carried out which were not to the benefit of individual patients but which wouldn't cause them significant harm and would benefit others. Since no harm can be done to the dead, this would mean PVS patients could be killed and their organs taken.

It is astonishing how far we've already travelled down this repellent road. The Law Commission report is on the shelf, but, like the proposal to allow "therapeutic" cloning, it will resurface when the public is softened up. The BMA's ethics division has succumbed to the same view that now clouds the vision of the Law Commission, health civil servants and most of the Establishment. It is the belief that nothing has intrinsic value and that the happiness of the greatest number trumps everything else.

Certain lives are thus expendable, and any objections are dismissed as religious, reactionary or loopy. We're supposed instead to cheer at this alliance between biotechnological big business and the government machine. . . . It is a moral universe where humanity itself has become no more than the sum of its body parts.

> "*The rationale for pursuing xenotransplantation [animal-to-human transplants] as a solution to the organ shortage is compelling.*"

Animal-to-Human Transplants Could Save Lives

John J. Fung

Numerous scientists have responded to the worsening organ shortage by exploring the possibilities of using animal organs for human transplants, a process known as xenotransplantation. In the following viewpoint, John J. Fung contends that research in xenotransplantation is critical because it may be a potential solution to the organ shortage. He suggests that technological advancements may be able to greatly lower the risks involved in xenotransplantations and could save many lives in the future. Fung is chief of transplantation at the University of Pittsburgh Medical Center.

As you read, consider the following questions:

1. Why is xenotransplantation becoming more clinically feasible, as stated by the author?
2. According to Fung, what are concordant and discordant xenotransplants?
3. In Fung's view, what is the major argument against xenotransplantation?

W ith the success of human-to-human transplantation, the need for organ replacement has grown to critical levels. (An estimated 65,000 Americans suffering from end-stage organ failure currently are awaiting organ transplantation and the number is growing each year.) The demand for organs has inspired concerted research efforts in the field of xenotransplantation—the use of animal organs as replacements for human organs. Nearly 5,000 people die each year because suitable donors are not found in time, so any progress toward expanding the pool of organs—including the use of animal organs—has implications that literally translate into human lives.

Clinically Feasible

Despite heightened public awareness to address the need for organ donation, there appears to be little prospect of increasing supplies to meet current shortages satisfactorily. The ability to use animal organs successfully as permanent replacements for failing human organs would end the suffering and death of patients awaiting transplantation. (More than 10% of patients awaiting transplantation die each year because of lack of human organs.) While artificial organs may become a reality with future developments, their ability to replace complex organs, such as the liver, is likely to be years away. Recent developments in understanding the barriers to successful xenotransplantation, along with access to novel drugs and approaches to manipulate the immune system, are making xenotransplantation more clinically feasible and bringing it much closer to reality.

Case reports of using animal kidneys appeared in the early 1900s from sources including pigs, goats, nonhuman primates, and lambs, but they met with failure, as did the earliest attempts at human-to-human transplantation. In the 1960s, a number of nonhuman primate-to-human kidney transplants were attempted, due to the pressing need for organs prior to the adoption of legislation that defined brain death and allowed cadaveric donation. Even with relatively ineffective forms of immunosuppression, function of non-human primate xenografts could be demonstrated, in one patient up to nine months after transplantation of a chimpanzee kidney.

In 1963, seven patients received baboon kidneys, all of which functioned immediately. These xenografts maintained dialysis-free function for up to 60 days before failing from rejection. With advances in immunosuppression and facing a severe shortage of pediatric donor hearts, Dr. Leonard Bailey transplanted a baboon heart into "Baby Fae" in 1983. Although that immunosuppressive regimen included cyclosporine, a new antirejection drug widely used today, the heart was eventually rejected 20 days after transplantation. No further attempts at xenotransplantation were done for almost a decade, until three attempts at liver xenotransplantation were reported between 1992 and 1993.

Concordant and Discordant Xenotransplants

When organs are transplanted across closely related species (e.g., baboon to human), such xenotransplants are referred to as "concordant." On the other hand, organs transplanted across widely divergent species (e.g., pig to human) are termed "discordant." These terms characterize the extent of difficulty that exists in striving for successful organ transplantation across these barriers. It is much easier to achieve xenograft acceptance across concordant than discordant combinations. Chimpanzees are considered the most biologically superior donor because they are genetically the closest to humans, but their threat of extinction precludes their use. Baboons, while not as similar to humans as chimpanzees, can be easily raised in captivity and are not an endangered species.

Pigs are available in sufficient quantities, have similar anatomy and physiology to humans, and can be bred under conditions in which they can be genetically modified. While these factors have prompted the consideration of this species as a source for clinical xenotransplantation, organs from discordant species are confronted with a formidable barrier—almost immediate rejection within minutes mediated by naturally occurring antibodies (also called preformed xenoantibodies) which are present in the recipient. Because of the difficulty in controlling such rejection (also known as hyperacute rejection), novel approaches are required to overcome this barrier to successful discordant xenotransplantation.

All humans have preformed antibodies to pig tissue, which would lead to hyperacute rejection of the transplanted xenograft. However, genetically modifying pigs—in essence, "humanizing" them—shows promise in preventing such a virulent rejection from taking place. A number of biotechnology companies and a handful of universities, including the University of Pittsburgh Medical Center, are taking a closer look at the potential this approach may yield for patients awaiting lifesaving organ transplants.

The Controversies of Xenotransplantation

What about the controversies surrounding the field of xenotransplantation? These are extensions of debates regarding broader issues of health care, biomedical research, organ transplantation, and human experimentation. The most recent discussions have focused on the possibility that infections from the donor would be transmitted to the human species. In the broadest sense, concern has been raised for society as a whole. It is the limited availability of data on the transfer of animal-derived, infectious pathogens to humans via xenotransplantation that has endangered the debate among scientists, physicians, regulatory agencies, and public representatives.

The scenario of unleashing a "doomsday" infectious agent on the human species has been forwarded by those who have urged a moratorium on xenotransplantation. The possibility of transmission of infectious agents following xenotransplantation certainly exists, since animals harbor infectious agents—such as bacteria, fungus, and parasites—that are known pathogens. These agents can be screened for, and, in most situations, effective therapy is available. Much less is known about the natural behavior of many human and animal viruses, let alone their singular or coexistent behavior in an organ recipient whose immune system is suppressed by the drugs needed to prevent organ rejection. Nevertheless, it is somewhat comforting that studies of diabetic patients who received pig pancreatic islet cells between four and seven years ago have had no evidence of pig-derived retroviruses, suggesting that the risk of this type of infection in these patients is small.

Nevertheless, it is the "unknown" agent that imparts caution in these trials. These unknown agents are either those that have not yet been identified or more hypothetically (and thus even scarier) "mutant" pathogens that might result from genetic recombination of human and animal viruses. This issue has been especially highlighted, in light of the putative origin of the human immunodeficiency virus (HIV), thought to arise from non-human primate cells.

A Twenty-First Century Answer

The era of xenotransplantation is here. . . . It is a twenty-first century answer to curing fatal diseases and prolonging life. Our society can no longer deny life-saving treatment to individuals simply because there are not enough human organs available. Xenotransplantation is a viable, exciting, and preferable option. The public will accept xenotransplantation better than the "presumed consent" system. Xenotransplantation may not fully replace human organs and tissue transplantation even with the recent successes of animal cloning. It can, however, serve as a back-up system for human graft donors. . . . We must be open to xenotransplantation as an alternative method that can eliminate the current human organ supply and demand problem.

Barbara Claxon-McKinney, *Pediatric Nursing*, September 2000.

In the past few years, the Food and Drug Administration, the Centers for Disease Control, and the National Institutes of Health have carefully reviewed the issues surrounding xenotransplantation. In early 1998, a special symposium was convened to develop guidelines for xenotransplantation trials. This conference called for the creation of a national Xenotransplantation Advisory Committee—comprised of scientists, physicians, ethicists, lawyers, and public representatives—to review public safety issues, using guidelines established by the transplant community for monitoring of infectious complications following clinical xenotransplant efforts. In addition, recommendations were made regarding the makeup of investigative teams at specialized centers that planned to embark on xenotransplantation trials.

The criticism surrounding xenotransplantation is strongly reminiscent of that leveled against human-to-human transplantation in the late 1960s and early 1970s. Yet, with persistence, the field of human-to-human transplantation has proven highly successful. This was the result of stepwise increases in understanding of the biology of rejection, improvements in drug management, and experience. Despite the resources that have been expended in efforts to promote human organ donations and given the unlikelihood of societal acceptance of mandated donation, the rationale for pursuing xenotransplantation as a solution to the organ shortage is compelling.

It is possible that xenotransplantation may not be universally successful until further technological advances occur, yet cautious exploration of xenotransplantation appears warranted, in order to identify those areas that require further study. Technological advances and better screening tools are likely to identify donors that may harbor latent infections or allow design of genetically engineered animals that may not be as susceptible to rejection or free from infectious risks. In addition, the principles learned from these early clinical cases possibly to utilize animal organs because of their innate resistance to infection or to peculiar species-specific metabolic pathways some day may lead to functional "cures" for diseases that prove resistant to other medical or surgical therapies. The use of animal organs may be the only way we can save more lives.

> *"There are serious financial and health consequences to xenografts [animal-to-human transplants]."*

Animal-to-Human Transplants Are Dangerous

Alan Berger and Gil Lamont

In the following viewpoint, Alan Berger and Gil Lamont contend that animal-to-human organ transplants, or xenotransplants, carry serious health consequences and should not be pursued. Berger and Lamont maintain that xenotransplants may infect humans with harmful viruses and that eliminating the dangers of viral infections across species may be impossible. The authors promote efforts to increase organ donation and encourage preventing illness through good diet and exercise. Berger is executive director of the Animal Protection Institute (API). Lamont is managing editor of *Animal Issues*, API's quarterly magazine.

As you read, consider the following questions:

1. How do Berger and Lamont support their view that xenotransplantation would be highly profitable?
2. According to the authors, what are the best-known diseases that have crossed from animals to humans?
3. In the authors' opinion, how may the shortage of organs be solved?

M ore than at any time in history, many of us today have the opportunity to live longer and healthier lives. Significant advances in immunosuppression and other techniques have greatly increased the success of human-to-human transplants ("allografts") to replace worn-out body organs. Too bad there aren't enough body parts to go around.

Despite encouraging organ donors—even the Department of Health and Human Services has a web site devoted to the issue at "http://www.organdonor.gov"—the number of waiting recipients is climbing steadily. In 1988, the United Network for Organ Sharing (UNOS) listed 16,026 registrants waiting for transplants. Today the list numbers nearly 55,000.

The number of donor organs, although increasing, has not kept pace. The pesky lack of donors has the medical community looking longingly at xenografts (animal-to-human transplants) as the perfect answer.

Good for Industry

Even when we put aside the serious ethical considerations of using animals as walking containers of spare parts, there are serious financial and health consequences to xenografts.

The wholesale adoption of xenotransplants, using organs from genetically altered pigs, will generate enormous profits for the pharmaceutical industry, for the bioengineering firms that supply the pigs, and for the medical professionals involved.

"Xenotransplantation," reports . . . [Judith Graham], "could become a $3 billion to $5 billion a year business within the next dozen years."

Good for industry, bad for the consumer. Already 40 million Americans are uninsured, increasing to 48 million—by 20%—in the year 2000. Another 29 million are underinsured.

Meanwhile, health care costs are skyrocketing. We spend $425 billion a year—two-thirds of all medical expenditures—to treat the six leading chronic diseases that cause nearly three-quarters of all deaths: heart disease, cancer, stroke, diabetes, obstructive pulmonary disease, and liver disease.

Current transplant costs range from $116,000 for a kidney to more than $300,000 for a liver. Factoring in five years of follow-up charges puts the costs at nearly $400,000 for a liver transplant, with heart, heart-lung, and lung transplants totaling more than $300,000 each. Adding xenografts to allografts will boost annual transplant expenditures from nearly $3 billion to $20.3 billion. And it can only rise from there.

Dwindling Confidence, Dwindling Coverage

Meanwhile, people's confidence in our health care system is dwindling. In a National Coalition on Health Care poll, 80% believe something is "seriously wrong" with the system and 87% believe that the quality of care needs to be improved. Eight of 10 blamed the profit motive for compromising quality.

"In these times of managed care and a nationwide glut of hospital beds," reported *The Wall Street Journal* on the reluctance of state officials to authorize $300 million to overhaul an aging hospital in Brooklyn, "reviving [these ailing medical centers] may make little economic sense. Experts say it is time for a better way: lean clinics that provide outpatient and primary care."

But when health care management takes services away from poorer neighborhoods, the "nationwide glut of hospital beds" is not available to the people who need them most, as revealed in a new study by the Harvard University School of Public Health. There's virtually no access to health care for native Americans on reservations, for urban blacks, for the poor concentrated anywhere. For them, health is poorer, life is shorter. Health care access can vary life expectancies by as much as 15 years between areas as little apart as 12 miles.

In a 1993 Kaiser/Commonwealth Fund health insurance survey, 34% of the uninsured reported that they failed to receive needed care, and 71% postponed needed care. And the uninsured who have chronic illnesses "are least likely to receive proper maintenance and continuous care, with the result that untreated conditions such as hypertension or diabetes can lead to serious health consequences."

Problem? What Problem?

Instead of allocating health costs to providing care to the millions who can't get it, our "baby boomer" bias concentrates on keeping that aging population bulge alive. Xenotransplant proponents have already begun a carefully orchestrated education of the public to accept xenografts, as evidenced by a recent press release [from the National Kidney Foundation]: "Nearly all Americans (94%) are aware of the shortage of available organs for transplant and most (62%) accept the concept of xenotransplantation, or animal-to-human transplantation, as a viable option." And "nearly 75 percent of people in all the groups surveyed would consider a xenotransplant for a loved one if the organ or tissue were unavailable from a human."

Evidently these people don't have all the facts. Certain diseases jump from animals to humans (zoonosis). The best known example is probably AIDS, which even Centers for Disease Control (CDC) scientists now acknowledge "resulted from the adaptation of simian retroviruses introduced across species lines into humans." The historically best known example is that of the 1918 influenza epidemic, which killed more than 20 million people worldwide and is now believed to have been a mutated swine virus carried to Europe by U.S. troops.

Nor are these isolated examples. Recently health officials in Hong Kong destroyed millions of chickens after a virus, A(H5N1), jumped directly from the birds to humans. And lately there has been much publicity over the occurrence of Creutzfeldt-Jakob disease (CJD), a fatal brain-wasting illness that has claimed a number of British humans' lives and which has been linked to mad cow disease (bovine spongiform encephalopathy).

No Getting Away from Viruses

The animal of choice for supplying xenotransplant organs is the pig. The transgenic pigs will be raised in a sterile environment, but pigs bring a whole new set of problems to the issue of xenosis (viruses transmitted during xenotransplants).

Recent findings by London researchers—at the Institute of Cancer Research and the National Institute of Medical Research (NIMR)—suggest that breeding virus-free pigs will be extremely difficult, if not impossible.

Sensitive molecular probes searched pigs from a range of breeds for copies of two inherited retroviruses, PERV-A and

PERV-B (porcine endogenous proviruses), which can infect human cells. All the pigs tested possessed multiple copies of the viruses, 10–23 copies of the PERV-A genes and 7–12 copies of PERV-B genes.

"The existence of 20 to 30 copies per cell will make it very much harder to remove the viruses from pig cells," said Dr. Jonathan P. Stoye of the NIMR, who led the research. "It may actually be impossible."

Blurring Ethical Boundaries

Opportunities exist to make medical breakthroughs by overcoming species' immune barriers in ways that blur ethical boundaries. The *British Medical Journal* recently published a letter on xenotransplantation from Neville Goodman, a physician. He is outraged that expensive high technology treatments like this are going forward at a time when political will is lacking to make basic medical resources available in the third world. With indignation, he quotes a researcher raising baboons for xenotransplant organs, who says her baboons "are treated better than some people in third world countries," as if proper treatment of the monkeys ends any ethical questions about xenotransplantation. "It seems that scientists are unclear and in profound disagreement among themselves as to where the lines should be drawn."

Margaret A. Clark, *Journal of Law, Medicine, and Ethics,* Summer 1999.

In the lab both viruses infect human cells, but nobody will commit to whether they will cause disease in people. Dr. Stoye, who wants further investigation before proceeding with pig-to-human xenotransplants, says, "We ought to know more about the pathogenic potential of these viruses."

We do know that humans can already acquire approximately 25 diseases from pigs, including anthrax, influenza, scabies, rabies, leptospirosis (which produces liver and kidney damage) and erysipelas (a skin infection).

Forging Ahead

Despite the above recognition that the dangers are unknown; despite the federal government's own assessment that the risk of infection cannot be quantified ("unequivocally greater than zero" was the official position); despite the requests of leading scientists that a moratorium be imposed on clinical xenotransplantation "in the public interest"; the government is committed to xenotransplantation.

At a December 1997 meeting, the Xenotransplant Advisory Subcommittee of the U.S. Food and Drug Administration (FDA) recommended that the FDA approve "limited" human clinical trials for xenotransplantation.

"Developing U.S. Public Health Service [PHS] Policy in Xenotransplantation," a January 1998 government-sponsored conference announced the imminent release of final PHS Guidelines for Xenotransplantation to Protect Against Infectious Diseases. The oversight agency for xenotransplantation will be the FDA.

The government intends to protect the public through cumbersome procedures that include screening donor animals for known viruses, constant surveillance of xenotransplant recipients and their contacts, maintaining tissue and blood samples from donor animals and human recipients, and establishing national and local registries of xenograft patients.

Given the scope of xenotransplants expected, the number of patients will, most likely, quickly outstrip the capabilities of the necessary database. As for screening for known viruses, what about the unknown ones? In February 1998, Australian scientists discovered an unknown virus in pigs. It apparently came from a colony of fruitbats that lived nearby. Once it hit the piggery the virus attacked pig fetuses, which were either stillborn or had defects in the spinal cord and brain. It also infected two human workers, who recovered. "You can't screen for disease agents that you don't know about," said virologist Peter Kirkland.

And after the virus is discovered, what can we really do about it? HIV has been known for decades, yet worldwide the AIDS epidemic is getting worse.

A Better Way

Would xenografts even be an option if enough human donor organs were available? Recent advances point the way to greater compatibility of organ and recipient. The discoverer of a "facilitating cell" that helps stem cells engraft says that "universal organ transplants may be possible, which may alleviate the chronic shortage of organs [according to *NewsEdge*]."

That "chronic shortage" may also be reduced by a new National Organ and Tissue Donor Initiative, and new policies in several states. Beginning in 1995, Pennsylvania hospitals are required to notify the regional organ procurement organization upon each patient's death to determine potential for organ or tissue donation. This immediately increased referrals tenfold. An aggressive education program has also increased public awareness of the need for donors, especially for people renewing their driver's licenses; in the first year, more than 820,000 drivers chose to have "organ donor" printed on the front of their licenses beneath their photograph. Similar legislation has been enacted or is being considered in New Jersey, Maryland, and other states.

While applauding all efforts to encourage more people to become organ donors, the Animal Protection Institute (API) supports enacting a national Presumed Consent Law, which supports a growing majority of Americans expressing a willingness to donate their organs at death. This law would assume that, *unless expressed otherwise before death*, everyone is a potential organ donor upon his or her demise. (Provisions for minors and the infirm require parental or guardian consent.) An opposite wish may simply be communicated in writing.

The Best of All

While transplants may offer longer and healthier lives to the chronically ill, one form of "medicine" reigns supreme. "I really don't think transplantation is going to be the answer," says Charles Porter, a Missouri cardiologist. "It's going to be rehabilitation and prevention." Rep. Jim Moran, D-Va., agrees, pointing out that the nation spends far too much on curing illnesses and not enough trying to prevent them. "Prevention," he says, "is much less expensive and far more effective."

Indeed, most illnesses are preventable. Changes in diet and increasing exercise can reduce high blood pressure, heart attacks, and cancer. Yet most people behave as if their bodies are machines to be worn out, or that the medical community sees transgenic pigs as the mobile warehouses for spare parts. Of the enormous numbers of dollars spent on health care, only a fraction goes to prevention and control efforts—about 3% of most state public health departments' budgets. In 1994, over $287 million was spent at the state level on prevention efforts aimed at the six leading chronic diseases (heart disease, cancer, stroke, diabetes, chronic obstructive pulmonary disease, and chronic liver disease). This was approximately 0.07% of the estimated $425 billion spent annually to treat those same diseases, according to a CDC study.

Xenotransplantation is not the answer, despite all the rosy pictures overoptimistic researchers, genetic engineers, and pharmaceutical companies paint of readily available organs. Since 1994, API has been saying exactly that, in a series of position papers, arguments, and at government-sponsored conferences. We cannot continue to cure human lives by the wholesale taking of animal lives. We cannot continue to deny health care to others simply because where they live prevents that health care from being "cost effective." We must learn to take better care of each other, by becoming organ donors, and better care of ourselves, through diet and exercise.

Periodical Bibliography

The following articles have been selected to supplement the diverse views presented in this chapter. Addresses are provided for periodicals not indexed in the *Readers' Guide to Periodical Literature*, the *Alternative Press Index*, the *Social Sciences Index*, or the *Index to Legal Periodicals and Books*.

Mark F. Anderson — "The Prisoner as Organ Donor," *Syracuse Law Review*, March 2000.

Linda Bronsdon — "I Donated My Kidney to a Stranger," *Self*, February 2001.

Christian Century — "Body Shop," June 21, 2000.

Paul Engstrom — "Second Chances: Older Patients Are Breaking Through Barriers That Once Limited Access to Donated Organs," *Wall Street Journal*, October 22, 2001.

Ian Hutchinson — "The Ethics of Xenotransplantation," *Biological Sciences Review*, November 1999.

Fred Kirsch — "The Greatest Gift of All," *Parade*, June 10, 2001.

Los Angeles Times — "Donating Life," October 11, 2001.

Celeste McGovern — "Give the Gift of Lips," *Alberta Report*, May 22, 2000.

Brigid McMenamin — "Swap Meet," *Forbes*, June 12, 2000.

Susan Okie — "Organ Exchanges Push Boundaries: New Tactics to Attract Donors Raise Issues of Ethics and Altruism," *Washington Post*, June 9, 2001.

Cathy Pascual and Thomas H. Maugh III — "Pig Organs Could Imperil Lives," *Los Angeles Times*, August 17, 2000.

Guy Rundle — "The Auto-Vivisectors," *Arena Magazine*, December 2000.

Gale Scott — "From Pigs to People: Do the Potential Risks of Animal-to-Human Transplants Outweigh the Benefits?" *New York Times*, October 2, 2001.

Joseph P. Shapiro — "A Swap That Cuts the Wait," *U.S. News & World Report*, July 23, 2001.

Deborah L. Shelton — "Seeking the Kindness of Strangers," *American Medical News*, November 6, 2001.

CHAPTER 3

Are Reproductive Technologies Ethical?

Chapter Preface

On December 20, 1998, Nkem Chukwu, a Texas woman, delivered seven of the eight fetuses she was carrying by cesarean section. They were born three months premature and weighed between 10.3 oz. and 1 lb. 10 oz. The smallest baby died from heart and lung failure within days. Two weeks later, Chukwu delivered the eighth baby, a girl. Doctors gave the Chukwu babies a 92 percent chance of survival. Although the following weeks were excruciating, the remaining infants survived.

Chukwu gave birth to the world's first living set of octuplets, in the same year that Chris Collins delivered septuplets in Iowa. Both women acknowledged that they had undergone fertility treatments when they faced difficulties in becoming pregnant. In fact, the increasing rate of "higher order" multiple births, defined as the birth of three or more babies from one pregnancy, reflects the spreading use of fertility drugs.

Many doctors are highly concerned about multiple births. Compared to normal pregnancies, infants of multiple births face significantly higher rates of mortality and lifelong health complications because of their extremely low birth-weight. Some studies indicate that among infants delivered at less than 1.7 pounds—the common weight of children born in higher order multiple births—half suffer from functional impairments, such as blindness and mental retardation.

When a woman faces a higher order multiple birth, doctors suggest that she abort some of the fetuses in order to increase the babies' overall chances of survival and long-term health. But due to their religious convictions, Chukwu and Collins refused to abort any of the fetuses. Although one of Collins's septuplets died shortly and two suffer from disabilities, she claims to be "honored to be their parent." On the other hand, all of Chukwu's surviving infants escaped long-term complications and have become healthy children.

Various controversial reproductive technologies have fulfilled some infertile couples' dreams of becoming parents. In the following chapter, authors discuss whether or not these technologies push ethical boundaries.

"Why not endorse [reproductive technologies'] contribution to ameliorating involuntary childlessness, while criticizing their problematic aspects?"

Reproductive Technologies Are Ethical

Dion Farquhar

Dion Farquhar is author of *The Other Machine: Discourse and Reproductive Technologies*. In the following viewpoint, Farquhar rebuts feminists' arguments against the use of reproductive technologies. She argues that feminists' complete rejection of such technologies is unfair to infertile women. She acknowledges the argument that reproductive technologies may oppress women, but contends that these technologies offer many benefits, such as allowing single women, lesbians, and gay men to have their own children.

As you read, consider the following questions:
1. According to the author, what are the implications of removing reproduction from heterosexual sex and marriage?
2. In the author's view, why do some feminists demonize reproductive technologies?
3. How does Farquhar respond to the argument that reproductive technologies are a "quick fix" to infertility?

The question of whether reproductive technologies benefit or harm their users, providers, and society as a whole has become an important element of contemporary feminist debate. Reproductive technologies are the medical capability to remove human eggs and sperm from one set of bodies, perform operations on them, and return them to the same female body, place them in another female body, or cryopreserve them. In addition to removing fertilization from the interior of women's bodies and transferring it to the laboratory, reproductive technologies also remove male ejaculation from its endpoint in the female body, reducing it to masturbation in clinic bathrooms.

All reproductive technologies separate reproduction from heterosexual sex and marriage. Potentially, that separation makes reproduction possible for those outside of the traditional heterosexual couple, offering new democratic family and parenting options. Not only are new individuals conceived as a result of technology, but so are new family, kinship, and parenting practices. Assisting reproductive technologies are expanding and challenging traditional views of just who may mother (or parent) a child today. Single heterosexual women, lesbians, single men, gay couples, and older women have fought for, and won, access to medical treatment. As more and more nontraditional would-be parents use the technologies, the ironclad identification of "mothering" with biology, heterosexuality, or even women, no longer holds.

Although there are obvious social benefits to removing reproduction from its biological constraints, there are many feminists who take a passionately antitechnology position. I want to argue that because reproductive technologies are a growing part of the U.S. social, economic, and medical scene, the point is not to be for or against them, but to ask what contributions they might make to the realization of feminists' goals. Our choices are not either to reject the technology entirely or to celebrate it uncritically. Reproductive technology, like maternity, is neither entirely oppressive and exploitative nor all-empowering and fulfilling. A woman's relations to reproductive technologies will depend on many complex biographical and historical factors.

Antitechnology feminists such as Rita Arditti, Gena Corea, Andrea Dworkin, Janice Raymond, Robyn Rowland, Patricia Spallone, and others have produced a large body of literature opposing assistive reproductive technologies for their complicity with the western liberal medical models of "disease," their essential sexual objectification of women's bodies and reproductive capacities, and for their unkindness to and abuse of women's bodies. Some of the points made by the antitechnology feminists are important and useful: e.g., their critique of our culture's compulsory natalism and the endemic sexism and racism of the western medical model; their analysis of the problem of class (the high cost of using these technologies severely restricts access and encourages the exploitation of desperate donors); and their exposure of the fertility clinic's false claims and misleading statistics on success rates. The problem is that in demonizing the technology, these theorists preclude admitting any liberatory potential for these technologies, which sometimes do satisfy the desires of individuals to have children and may also expand our cultural understanding of family and kinship.

Ambivalence Toward Maternity

Underlying the demonization of technology that is evident in the opposition to assistive reproductive technologies is a radical ambivalence toward maternity. On the one hand, the antitechnology writing brims with an antinatalist stance that configures women's nurturance as unequivocally supportive of patriarchal domination. Women's desires for maternity are seen as the externally imposed burden of patriarchal ideology, a parasitic sapping of women's physical and emotional energies that deflects women's time and attention from more important aspects of public life—knowledge, power, money and so on. Antinatalists find the whole project of helping women reproduce and become either genetic or gestational mothers problematic because it reinforces the already near-compulsory cultural bias toward maternity. The only shift, according to this antinatalist vision, is that rather than being controlled by individual men through marriage, women will be controlled by science and technology. Childbearing in this view is either rejected or suffered.

The same antitechnology literature, however, sometimes glorifies motherhood as the apogee of care and nurturance, the basis for an alternative ethics, and the source of women-centered knowledge. This pronatalist stance, though, is limited to "naturally" achieved maternity. Technological intervention is opposed on the grounds that it fragments unitary maternity, threatens to displace "natural" motherhood, and interferes in "natural" maternal processes. Pronatalist "natural" maternity is seen as unambiguously enriching to (all) women just as, for the antinatalists, maternity is seen as a patriarchal rip-off of (all) women's unpaid and unappreciated reproductive and emotional labor.

A Fuller Appreciation

In these times we are facing major decisions, both individually and as a society, in relation to our own reproduction. While scientific advances have provided hope to couples experiencing difficulty in having children they have simultaneously raised fundamental personal and communal questions about what it means to be human. The issues raised by these questions highlight the fact that, embedded within our shared humanity lie certain principles which cannot be ignored in ethical decision-making. The growth of assisted reproductive technologies tends to outstrip our ability to fully appreciate the ethical and moral implications of their use. We believe that an understanding of moral and ethical principles will allow us individually and collectively to make informed judgements about the use of assisted human reproductive technologies. These principles are derived from our understanding of what it means to be fully human and to live in community.

To assist in this understanding we outline principles which require consideration in any use of assisted reproductive technologies: respect for the dignity of human life; protection of the vulnerable; respect for autonomy; informed consent; the balancing of individual and collective interests; the right to genetic information and knowledge of origins. It is our belief that these principles provide a framework through which the stability and integrity of society can be promoted as we move towards a fuller appreciation of the implications of the use of these technologies.

New Zealand Catholic Bishops' Conference, "Statement on Assisted Human Reproductive Technologies," 1998.

This contradictory discourse forces antitechnology feminists to invoke "false consciousness" to explain (mostly) middle-class white women's escalating demands for high-technology infertility services: "But sometimes women also collude because we have been brainwashed. The information and education we get is one-sided and male-centered and the hidden conviction creeps into our own minds that men and their technology must be better than our own body and our own experiences with it," writes Renate Duelli Klein. Reproductive technologies all "violate the integrity of a woman's body in ways that are dangerous, destructive, debilitating, demeaning; they are a form of medical violence against women," argues Janice Raymond in her latest book, *Women as Wombs*. For antitechnologists, the female "experience" is universal; there are no exceptions, no individuals for whom they do not speak.

Whether pronatalist, antinatalist, or both, antitechnologists basically displace feminist ambivalence toward motherhood onto the technologies themselves. As feminist writer Michelle Stanworth, in her article "Birth Pangs," has noted: "A focus on the degrading impact of conceptive technologies is attractive, perhaps, because it seems to make possible the impossible: to attack the coercive aspects of maternity, the way that motherhood makes victims of women—and to do so in the name of motherhood itself." In attacking technology, however, we hold infertile women to a higher standard of political purity, particularly since feminists have never successfully countered the pronatalist expectations of our society. Generally, we live in a culture in which "childlessness" is frowned upon and motherhood is still taken for granted.

The Technology Debate

A deep ambivalence about motherhood, however, is not the only reason that some feminists oppose reproductive technologies. Antitechnology feminists also write about the superficiality of the interventions. They assert that the high-tech medical treatment of infertility is a "quick fix" rather than a correction of underlying pathology. Prescribing in vitro fertilization (IVF) for the treatment of blocked, diseased, or absent fallopian tubes only bypasses them, providing a technological "fix" without ameliorating the underlying problem. Though this may be true, why should we necessarily feel that it is problematic to circumvent the malfunctioning part of the conception process, if this is the most direct route to bearing a child?

A related objection of antitechnology feminists to high-tech treatments is that they fail to address the underlying macro-epidemiological causes of infertility: environmental pollution, workplace toxicity, iatrogenic (inadvertently produced) factors, untreated or undiagnosed pelvic inflammatory disease, among others. Ignoring such epidemiological evidence, they argue, greedy high-technology promoters focus only on treating the individual once she or he is found to be infertile.

Both of these antitechnology arguments point out critical gaps in the medical and popular representations of reproductive technologies; they are entirely valid as social analyses. These criticisms, however, like all the others, excoriate the technologies for their individual focus and failure to address the social causes of infertility without providing any possibilities for infertile people. The antitechnology position suggests that infertile women, whose wills are porous ciphers of the patriarchy, should "choose" to forego the use of such technologies. As Gena Corea and Jalna Hanmer have written in the prologue to *Made to Order: The Myth of Reproductive and Genetic Progress*, "the desire of some individual women to 'choose' this technology place women as a group at risk. With the new reproductive technologies, women are being used as living laboratories and are slowly but surely being divorced from control over procreation."

This position endorses a reproductive double standard for infertile people, approving, albeit idealizing, those who reproduce "naturally" and opposing the use of technology as pronatalist for those who experience physical or social obstacles. The imposition of a strict, politically pure double standard on infertile people who wish to use such technologies is like blaming cancer patients for "choosing" individualist therapies like chemotherapy or radiation rather than campaigning for the reduction of pesticides or pollutants. Infertile people are no more or less responsible than the rest of the population for campaigning for a healthier environment or sterility prevention.

Here to Stay

Like many aspects of life in the contemporary United States, reproductive technologies are a mixed blessing. There seems no point in simply opposing them, since they are here to stay. Moreover, why not endorse their contribution to ameliorating involuntary childlessness, while criticizing their problematic aspects? Reproductive technologies have the potential to change radically the nature of family and kinship. As feminists, we should seek to expand women's access to these technologies, to regulate the provision of services, and to build a social movement that addresses environmental causes of male and female sterility and infertility.

> "Technological reproduction has made
> medicalised access to the female body
> acceptable, and medicalised abuse . . .
> 'for our own good.'"

Reproductive Technologies Are Unethical

Janice G. Raymond

Janice G. Raymond is a professor of women's studies and medical ethics at the University of Massachusetts at Amherst and author of *Women as Wombs: Reproductive Technologies and the Battle over Women's Freedom*. In the following viewpoint, Raymond contends that reproductive technologies are invasive and endanger women's health. She maintains that the medical profession has defined infertility as a medical problem in order to justify the use of harmful, ineffective technologies that exploit women's bodies.

As you read, consider the following questions:
1. How does Raymond support her argument that the medical profession has established a misleading definition of infertility as a medical problem?
2. According to Raymond, how has the medical profession responded to the perceived problem of fertility in the Third World?
3. What is the author's view of surrogacy?

From "Reproduction, Population, Technology, and Rights," by Janice G. Raymond, *Women in Action*, www.isiswoman.org, February 1998. Copyright © 1998 by Women in Action. Reprinted with permission.

This viewpoint will address the globalisation of new reproductive technologies and drugs and, as a framework for this discussion, the industrialisation of reproduction.

It is the reproduction of fertility and infertility with which I am concerned, i.e., the ways in which both fertility and infertility are being created and commodified as medically managed problems by medicine, media, and commerce. When the "disease" of infertility is established, what follows is the deployment of distinctively different technologies developed for use in different parts of the world.

Programs and policies supporting new reproductive technologies are governed by ideologies of fertility and infertility.

In the industrialized countries of the North, it is infertility that is being produced and marketed by those who would tell us that infertility rates are skyrocketing. Infertility is the new frigidity, and technology is the new instrumental manipulation that will coax reluctant women's bodies into reproductive performance. Technological reproduction has made medicalised access to the female body acceptable, and medicalised abuse—that a woman will endure anything to become pregnant—standard treatment "for our own good."

The Problem of Infertility

Is there a real problem of infertility in the Northern countries?

Certainly, infertility caused by environmental pollution and sexually transmitted diseases (STDs), as well as medically-induced infertility such as pelvic inflammatory disease (PID) caused by IUDs, is on the rise. The media and infertility experts talk about an epidemic of infertility in the North with one out of six or seven couples being infertile. Yet both the National Centre for Health Statistics (NCHS) and the U.S. Office of Technology Assessment (OTA) contend that the more accurate figure is one in twelve. What has expanded is the definition of infertility.

Although infertility is a concept that has no scientific consensus, the currently accepted medical definition is inability to conceive after one year of intercourse without contraception. The number of years has dwindled in recent times, from five to two to one. Thus the definition conflates inability to conceive with difficulty in conceiving quickly. This routes a large number of women into unnecessary, experimental and costly medical treatment all the sooner.

The media portrayal of infertility and the infertile is deceptively simple and homogeneous. Those undergoing in vitro fertilization (IVF), for example, are portrayed as forever infertile. Yet a large percentage have had children in a present or a previous relationship. Many women undergo IVF because their husbands are infertile. This is probably one of the only examples in medical practice where a proxy is treated, i.e., another undergoes procedures in place of the actual person with the problem. Percentages vary, but it has been estimated that 11–35 percent of women on IVF programs are there because of male partners' problems. Male-factor infertility is as common as female factor, yet often the male partner is not tested in infertility assessments, or only after the woman has undergone extensive and exhaustive evaluation. Women testify that many gynecologists never order analysis of their husbands' sperm. And frequently, men will not undergo the tests, viewing them as offensive to their virility. Because women undergo the IVF procedures, many men are spared the embarrassment of having their infertility known. . . .

The Problem of Fertility

In the developing countries of the South, Northern population agencies use a different rationale for promoting new reproductive techniques and drugs.

Here, it is fertility that is the perceived problem. The consequences of technological reproduction to women in developing countries have been sterilization and use of new/old and dangerous contraceptive implants, injectables, and antipregnancy vaccines. The pill was initially tried on women in Puerto Rico. The Dalkon shield, an IUD taken off the market in most First World countries, remains implanted in many Third World women. Third World countries have long been a dumping ground for chemicals and drugs such as DDT banned in the industrialised countries.

Women in Brazil and Bangladesh were among the first tested in Norplant trials. Norplant is the contraceptive implant that remains embedded under a woman's skin for about five years. It generated such problems in Brazilian women—dramatic change in body weight, heavy bleeding and menstrual irregularities, and severe alterations of the central nervous system—the feminist groups, in cooperation with a government study committee, succeeded in cancelling the trials—for a time. Yet when Norplant was approved by the United States Drug Administration (FDA) for use in the United States, the Brazilian data was not evident.

The rationale of female-fertility-out-of-control-in-the-Third-World has generated another and more drastic "treatment"—sex predetermination. Women have long been viewed as the cause of population proliferation in developing countries and, for the last 25 years, some scientists have proposed that by reducing the number of women born, the so-called population problem would be solved.

Sex Predetermination Goals

In India especially, massive termination of female pregnancies has been achieved by abortion after amniocentesis reveals the sex of the foetus. Between 1978 and 1983, almost 80,000 female foetuses were aborted there. Given the overwhelming preference for male children, the maltreatment of girl children, and the punishment meted out to women who do not produce sons, it is not surprising that, as the rationale goes, women "ask for" the technology.

A U.S. entrepreneur of sperm separation technology—Ronald Ericsson of Gametrics, Inc.—has set up a chain of clinics in India, Jordan, Pakistan, Egypt, Malaysia, Singapore, and Taiwan, as well as several in the United States. Pivet, a west Australian company, has established in vitro fertilisation clinics in Brazil, India, Malaysia, and Indonesia, partially for sex predetermination goals. Clinics have been deluged with requests from financially well-off women both affected by infertility but also by the stigma of not having produced a son. Pivet is a prime example of a company developing a technology (IVF) usually used to promote fertility that, in a developing country context, is used quite differently to prevent fertility.

In the industrialised countries of the North, in vitro fertilisation is the basis for all the rest of the technologies. Once egg and sperm are placed in a petri dish, researchers and clinicians determine the sex of the embryo, freeze eggs and embryos, transfer the embryo from one woman to another, or use the embryos for experimentation and genetic manipulation. Initially looked upon as a "fringe" technology, today IVF is regarded as the most conservative of new reproductive procedures.

Over 200 U.S. institutions performing IVF treatment have been established in the last decade. In the absence of federal funds for research in this area, the tab has been picked up by patients, pharmaceutical companies, universities and hospitals, and private organisations often relying on venture capitalism. A large number of these centers are for-profit "fertility institutes" that perform other reproductive services such as surrogacy and sex predetermination as well. Although rates vary, a conservative figure that clients pay is about $5,000 per IVF cycle. Many women return for two, five, and sometimes 10 cycles.

The United States, however, is not the reproductive technology capital of the world. France and Australia compete for this title. For example, France has more IVF centers per capita than any other country in the world; Australia has had the highest success rates and an infusion of government spending for the technologies. Australia has exported its IVF technology to the United States in a venture known as IVF Australia which has set up many for-profit fertility centers in this country, as well as in Europe and many developing countries.

A Rapidly Expanding Market

Despite the absence of federal monies in the United States, the technological reproduction market is expanding rapidly. Groups of doctors have joined the entrepreneurial fray here and have helped spawn a rapid proliferation of new drugs and technologies. For example, doctors who own Northern Nevada Center, an IVF clinic, believe that eventually IVF could be a $6 billion annual business.

Rarely has a technology with such a dismal success rate been so quickly accepted. Half of the clinics in the United States reporting success had never had a live birth. Definitions of pregnancy varied widely (you thought you knew one when you saw one, but not in the realm of IVF statistics). In a statistical sleight of hand, some centers claimed success by the number of completed implantations that never resulted in births, or by the number of chemical pregnancies (elevation of hormone level that may but often doesn't indicate an ongoing pregnancy). Even some of the IVF experts admitted that "it's not easy to fudge results."

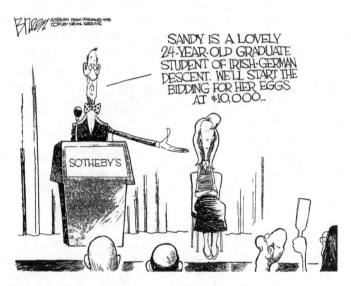

Breen. © 1999 by Copley Media Services. Reprinted with permission.

In fact, IVF's very lack of success has been the justification for developing new technical variations of IVF (such as GIFT and TUDOR) as well as superovulation and embryo freezing. Doctors argued for embryo freezing to reduce the number of egg retrievals, and thus the trauma to the ovaries caused by multiple inductions of ovulation. They also claimed that superovulation—medical sorties of powerful fertility drugs used to blast the ovaries into multiple egg production—would enable clinicians to "capture" eggs not accessible to laparoscopy.

More recently, the problems created by superovulation and multiple implants of fertilized eggs into a woman's uterus, i.e., multiple foetuses, have been used to justify foetal reduction—

or in its kinder and gentler idiom, "selective termination of pregnancy." Doctors inject a saline solution into the uterus to abort a certain number of foetuses. This technique can cause bleeding, danger of premature labor, and even the loss of foetuses. There is a concern also about damage to any foetuses that remain.

With the infinite expansionism of technological reproduction—IVF, embryo transfer, embryo freezing, and the use of fertility drugs—medicine inflates the perceived "need" for newer technologies to solve the complications caused by the older procedures. Has faith in medical progress reached the point where people accept, without criticism, the reality that last technological "mistakes" need more technological solutions which themselves turn into problems? If so, this is the height of technological determinism.

A Form of Medical Violence

When technologies harm foetuses and children, people take note—but not when the harm occurs to women.

What has been most invisible in the whole debate over new reproductive technologies worldwide is the harm that accrues to women and which, in reality, could be viewed as a form of medical violence against women: hyperstimulation of the ovaries and possible cysts resulting from superovulation, along with the pain and trauma of the entire IVF process itself. There have also been at least 10 deaths of women that have been connected with IVF procedures.

Traditional morality has challenged these technologies from a foetal-centered perspective, but not from the viewpoint of feminist ethics which is woman-centered. Many ethicists, scientists and policy-makers are worried about the quality of life—the humanity—of so-called test tube babies. Feminist critics are primarily concerned with the quality of life of women who submit to being used as "living laboratories" of reproduction. Traditional ethics is preoccupied with experimentation on foetuses; feminists have consistently pointed out that the primary experimentation in this realm is on women. Would that women enjoyed the same respect and dignity that foetuses get in the halls of traditional morality and law.

Surrogacy

Then there is surrogacy, or contract pregnancy. In this situation, a woman bears a child for another person or couple and gives over the child at birth to be raised by the contracting party. In the United States, the surrogate industry has brokered many contract pregnancies that for the most part have been looked upon as an individual arrangement between an altruistic woman (usually one who needs money) and a couple who is supposedly desperate to have a child.

But others view surrogacy as reproductive purchase orders where women are procured as instruments in a system of commercial breeding. It is more accurate, in this view, to call surrogacy reproductive trafficking because it creates a national and international traffic in women in which women become moveable property, objects of reproductive exchange, and brokered by go-betweens mainly serving the buyer.

There are many women in the United States hired as surrogates who now speak out against this reproductive servitude. Beyond the reality of "regular" surrogacy is "pure" surrogacy involving women who contribute no egg but do the "mere" carrying to term. In 1990, Anna Johnson, an African-American, bore a child for Mark Calvert, a Euro-American man, and his Asian-American wife, Christina Calvert. Before Johnson delivered the baby, she announced her intention to fight for custody in court. But the California court awarded all parental rights to the gamete providers—the ejaculatory father and the egg mother—and in so doing, affirmed that genetics was the primary criterion of parenthood.

Feminists predicted the exploitation of Anna Johnson about 10 years ago in warning that surrogate brokers and contracting individuals would seek out "pure" surrogates from women of color since, at that point, the skin color wouldn't matter. Yet in surrogate gestation where the so-called surrogate contributes her egg, there is an insidious way in which skin color is exactly what does matter. It was the blackness of Anna Johnson's skin that worked against her legal claim to the light-skinned child.

Indeed surrogate brokers have frankly admitted that they will turn to Third World women for their stables of contract breeders. There, brokers maintain, the going rate will be cheaper and the labour supply more submissive. John Stehura, president of the Bionetics Foundation, talked about his plans for a surrogate business in Mexico that would use local women for U.S. clients. In an interview with Gena Corea, Stehura maintained that "You could devastate them (Mexican women) with money and things. . . . It would save them 20 years of scratching."

The specter of international reproductive exploitation has become so serious that the vulnerability of women in developing countries at risk for surrogacy, or "womb renting" has been raised at various committee hearings overseeing the Convention to Eliminate All Forms of Discrimination Against Women (CEDAW). . . .

There is [an] unwillingness today to recognize the magnitude of reproductive violations. Unrecognized is the creation of a new form of the international medical research networks; the technology transfers; the global markets for surrogacy which follow established international adoption routes; the expanding international demand for and supply of foetal tissue, eggs, embryos for medical research; the international stockpiling of frozen embryos. Dr. Fritz Hondlus, deputy director of legal affairs for the Council of Europe, reported that as of 1989, over 200,000 embryos were stored in Europe alone because, as he characterised it, IVF practice was out of control in European clinics.

The Biological Laboratory of the Future

All reproductive technologies and arrangements are a political issue. They are an indication of the power or lack of power that women have over our bodies. And they are an indication of the degree to which access to the female body has become as normative in the reproductive realm, as it has been in the sexual realm. The image of women as reproductive objects, as sexual objects, is fast becoming reality.

Portrayed as medical miracles by the media, we must ask why these medical miracles require that women adapt to painful and debilitating intervention.

Why are women channeled, at such a cost to their bodies and themselves, into reproducing children for themselves and for others? Or, as is the case in many developing countries, why are women routed into not reproducing by state mandate or incentive programs that promote more risky and harmful methods such as Norplant, DepoProvera and the vaccines? In many countries, why is it that women who want safe and adequate contraception have difficulty obtaining it when religion and the state combine to legislate women's reproductive options? Why do these techniques reinforce the biomedical view that a woman's reproductive system is pathological and requires an enormous amount of intervention?

Under the cover of a new science of reproduction, is the female body being fashioned into the biological laboratory of the future?

*"Surrogacy, as a family-building option,
implicates . . . procreative freedom."*

Surrogate Motherhood Is Ethical

Lawrence A. Kalikow

Surrogate motherhood, in which a woman either volunteers or is paid to carry the embryo of another couple until birth, has allowed couples faced with fertility challenges to have their own children. In the following viewpoint, Lawrence A. Kalikow claims that surrogate motherhood helps couples to assert their procreative freedom. Kalikow argues that the majority of surrogacy arrangements are successful and contribute to the happiness and prosperity of many families. The author urges that surrogacy be protected so that it remains a "family-building option" for infertile couples. Kalikow is a lawyer in North Wales, Pennsylvania.

As you read, consider the following questions:
1. In the author's opinion, what are the limitations of adoption?
2. According to Kalikow, what are the typical characteristics of couples that seek surrogacy arrangements?
3. What did the California Supreme Court rule on the issue of commercial surrogacy in the *Calvert* case?

From "Why Legislators Should Pass Positive Legislation Regarding Surrogacy," by Lawrence A. Kalikow, www.opts.com, September 2, 1997. Copyright © 1997 by the Organization for Parents Through Surrogacy, Inc. Reprinted by permission of the author.

From time immemorial, oppressive governments have banned or imposed undue restrictions on everything from religious practices to books largely because of ignorance and lack of respect for individual liberty. Attempts to control human reproduction—such as the perverse restrictions devised by Nazi Germany more than a half century ago and the draconian measures more recently imposed by Communist China—are a particularly odious form of governmental intrusion into the most intimate of all human affairs, the decision to have a child.

We, as a nation with a history and constitutional framework evincing unparalleled respect for individual rights and liberties, should be loath to embark on a path of state-imposed restrictions treading on the right of privacy and procreative freedom.

Surrogacy, as a family-building option, implicates both the right of privacy and procreative freedom. Recognition of the foregoing was eminently well expressed by a number of distinguished state senators from Pennsylvania, who in 1991, co-sponsored a surrogate parenting bill that expressly set forth the following finding:

> . . . an individual's decision regarding whether or not to bear or beget a child falls within the constitutionally protected right of privacy, and, therefore, the Commonwealth may not prohibit the practice of surrogate parenting or enact regulations that would have the effect of prohibiting that practice.

In order to properly understand surrogacy, one must first have an understanding of infertility. Few things can touch an adult human being more intimately or affect him or her more pervasively than the inability to have a child. The psychological and emotional consequences can be devastating. Infertility often consumes those afflicted by it, leaving in its wake emptiness, grief and despair. Those who have been blessed with children can only imagine the deep void that would exist in their lives without them.

Pro-Family and Pro-Life

While conventional adoption may be a viable alternative for some infertile couples, there are significant limitations with adoption as a family-building option. For many couples, age restrictions, costs, the limited number of adoptable children (particularly healthy newborns) and the prospect of a protracted emotional "roller coaster" may effectively foreclose adoption. Moreover, conventional adoption will not result in a genetically related child. Often, surrogacy alone provides that possibility. The desire to have a genetically related child is deeply rooted in the human psyche and should be neither condemned nor denigrated. Undeniably, few couples of the fertile world would choose to forego having their own genetic offspring in favor of adoption.

Surrogacy is clearly consistent with and, indeed, furthers deeply held societal values. Because it is the very means through which an infertile couple brings a child into the world, surrogacy is inherently pro-family and is, in the truest sense, emphatically pro-life. Properly done, surrogacy is a carefully structured collaborative creative effort that holds the potential for great joy and happiness and for the development of a unique and truly wonderful set of human relationships. Few of our social institutions—indeed, few human endeavors—can boast a success rate approximating that of surrogacy. Of thousands of surrogate parenting arrangements that have been entered into, only a small handful (far fewer than one percent) have resulted in litigation over custody. The vast majority are glowing success stories. Unfortunately, however, such happy outcomes are not likely to make their way to prime time television.

That surrogacy is so successful as a family-building option is not surprising. Most couples who choose to pursue surrogacy do so only after lengthy infertility treatment, followed by careful study and reflection. Many receive some form of counseling or other professional guidance even before embarking on the process. Overwhelmingly, those intending to parent through surrogacy are in stable, long-term marriages and are responsible, law abiding and productive members of society. Above all else they share an intense desire to have a child and become a family. Surrogacy is rarely undertaken without extensive preparation, screening and planning. Indeed, the typical surrogate parenting arrangement involves far more medical and psychological screening prior to achieving a pregnancy than does conventional conception or conventional adoption and includes a comprehensive written agreement, memorializing the intentions, as well as the respective obligations, of the intended parents and the surrogate mother. Hence, in a very real sense surrogacy is the ultimate in planned parenthood.

The Perceived Problem

The perceived problem with surrogacy is one largely created by distorted, sensationalized media coverage of a few aberrational cases and by some bioethicists, cloistered in ivory towers and insulated from real life experience. It is clearly anomalous to judge surrogate parenting based upon its very few failures. Surely, no one can seriously maintain that conventional adoption ought to be condemned because so many adoptions ultimately fall through or that marriage ought to be condemned because of a growing incidence of spouse abuse or a spiraling divorce rate. Measured against any objective standard—and, especially, when compared with other practices and institutions—surrogate parenting has not posed a significant problem in any state. . . .

In the absence of an amply demonstrated compelling need to rectify an actual rather than a perceived problem, lawmakers should shun legislation that intrudes upon the right of privacy and curtails procreative freedom. While legislatively imposed restrictions on any human activity always exact a price in terms of diminished freedom and narrowed choices, the price exacted by banning or unduly restricting surrogate parenting will for many of those affected be tragically high: the dream of having a child and becoming a family. Wisdom and compassion, as well as sensitivity to the constitutional rights implicated, dictate a different approach.

Presently, the majority of states have not enacted laws that ban or severely restrict surrogate parenting. Typically, those states that have enacted such laws have done so as a visceral, knee-jerk response in the wake of New Jersey's Baby M case. [In the Baby M case, a surrogate mother unsuccessfully sought full custody of a child she bore through artificial insemination for another couple in a surrogacy contract.] While no legislation is far better than draconian restrictions, legislation that preserves surrogacy as a viable family-building option, that is sensitive to the constitutional issues, practical concerns and human feelings involved and that establishes certainty with respect to legal parentage is a laudable goal. Any legislation in this complex area, however, should not result from precipitant action based upon ill-informed beliefs inflamed by distorted and sensationalized media coverage of the most aberrational cases. Rather, it should be the product of careful, laborious study, with input sought from those truly knowledgeable about surrogate parenting.

Problems and Complications

Even if commercial surrogate motherhood (C.S.M.) is not immoral, perhaps it should be illegal? Perhaps, as its opponents suggest, it should be illegal because of the problems it can and could create?

Various things in life cause problems and complications. This is not in itself much of an argument for making them crimes. For instance, marriage causes complications and problems as does having, even in the normal way, children. How many people regret having married and/or regret having had children (or regret not having had children)? Plenty of them. Should marriage on that account be made illegal? Should the having of children (or the failure to have children) become criminal offences? Hardly.

Hugh V. McLachlan and J.K. Swales, *Contemporary Review*, March 1998.

Any legislation that would prohibit the payment of compensation would have a devastating impact upon surrogacy: it would effectively foreclose surrogacy as a lawful family-building option for most couples. Moreover, criminalizing the payment of compensation would inevitably make criminals of otherwise honest, law-abiding, productive citizens, whose only "crime" would be attempting to create a biologically-related family. It would also cruelly stigmatize many children who have already been born of successful surrogacy arrangements that involved the payment of compensation.

Fair and Appropriate

Contrary to what some bioethicists have suggested, neither the payment nor acceptance of compensation for a surrogate mother's participation in a surrogate parenting arrangement can reasonably be viewed as the "buying" or "selling" of a baby. Particularly in light of the tremendous amount of time, energy and effort that the surrogate mother necessarily expends in any surrogate parenting arrangement, reasonable compensation is both fair and appropriate. Furthermore, the Supreme Court of California, in *Calvert v. Johnson*, (1993), and the Supreme Court of Kentucky, in *Surrogate Parenting Associates, Inc. v. Com. ex rel. Armstrong*, (1986), dealt explicitly with the compensation issue and emphatically rejected the arguments advanced by the opponents of surrogacy. Central to both decisions was the recognition that surrogacy is fundamentally different from conventional adoption. As the courts reasoned, unlike conventional adoption, surrogacy involves a preconception agreement that the surrogate will carry a child for the intended parents and, unlike conventional adoption, in every surrogate parenting arrangement at least one intended parent is a genetic parent of the child.

In ruling that the law prohibiting the buying and selling of children did not apply to surrogate parenting arrangements, the *Armstrong* court aptly observed:

> . . . the central fact in the surrogate parenting procedure is that the agreement to bear the child is entered into before conception. The essential considerations for the surrogate mother when she agrees to the surrogate parenting procedure are not avoiding the consequences of an unwanted pregnancy or fear of the financial burden of child rearing. On the contrary, the essential consideration is to assist a person or couple who desperately want a child but are unable to conceive one in the customary manner to achieve a biologically related offspring. The problem is caused by the wife's infertility. The problem is solved by artificial insemination. The process is not biologically different from the reverse situation where the husband is infertile and the wife conceives by artificial insemination.

Similarly, in upholding the surrogate parenting agreement in the case before it, the *Calvert* court stated:

> We are likewise unpersuaded by the claim that surrogacy will foster the attitude that children are mere commodities; no evidence is offered to support it. The limited data available seem to reflect an absence of significant adverse effects of surrogacy on all participants. The argument that a woman cannot knowingly and intelligently agree to gestate and de-

liver a baby for intending parents carries overtones of the reasoning that for centuries prevented women from attaining equal economic rights and professional status under the law. To resurrect this view is both to foreclose a personal and economic choice on the part of the surrogate mother, and to deny intending parents what may be their only means of procreating a child of their own genetic stock.

The sensitivity and wisdom reflected in the *Calvert* and *Armstrong* opinions should loom large in any consideration of the issues involved in surrogacy.

A Viable Family-Building Option

Although surrogacy is intensely important to those infertile couples who already have created a family through that option or who hope to do so in the future, it is clearly not viewed as an important issue by the vast majority of the electorate. Unlike so many problems, such as crime, teen pregnancy and child abuse, that do regularly adversely affect the general public, surrogacy has had virtually no discernable negative impact. Rather, it has provided the means through which some very good citizens have been able to fulfill the dream of creating a family.

Even in 1987, at the height of the adverse publicity surrounding the Baby M case, a *Newsweek* poll revealed that more than sixty (60%) percent of Americans had no problem with surrogacy provided that the intended mother could not herself conceive and/or carry a child. As the public learns more about infertility in general and surrogate parenting in particular, support for anti-surrogacy legislation is likely to continue to wane.

Far from benefitting anyone, the enactment of anti-surrogacy legislation is certain to cause grief and despair. Can anything be more devastating to flesh and blood human beings than the death of the dream of creating a family? Any lawmaker considering anti-surrogacy legislation should give ample thought to that question before casting his or her vote. On the other hand, sponsoring and/or supporting salutary legislation that preserves surrogate parenting as a viable family-building option can help others realize that dream and the great happiness that flows from it.

> "The main objection to commercial
> surrogacy is that it is the equivalent of
> baby selling, a practice that is inherently
> morally objectionable."

Surrogate Motherhood Is Unethical

Scott B. Rae

In the following viewpoint, Scott B. Rae contends that surrogate motherhood, in which one woman is impregnated with another couple's embryo to bear them a child, is unethical because it constitutes baby selling. Rae repudiates the argument that the surrogate mother is paid for her reproductive capacities. Instead, the payment is for the waiver of the surrogate mother's parental rights, which is morally objectionable. Rae is the author of several books on ethics, including *The Ethics of Commercial Surrogate Motherhood: Brave New Families?* from which this viewpoint is excerpted.

As you read, consider the following questions:

1. According to Rae, what are the various forms of the argument that surrogate mothers are paid for their gestational services, not the sale of a child?
2. In the author's opinion, what differences do surrogacy proponents see between surrogacy and black market adoptions?
3. What evidence does Rae provide for the potential commercial exploitation of women's reproductive systems?

In the *Baby M* case,[1] the New Jersey Supreme Court equated surrogacy with baby selling, in violation of the state's adoption laws. The lower court had maintained that surrogacy cannot be baby selling since one of the parties involved is the natural father. The lower court ruled that the adoption laws did not contemplate surrogacy arrangements, and thus that extending them to surrogacy was invalid. The state Supreme Court sharply disagreed, defining surrogacy as inherently the sale of children, rejecting any attempts to evade what the court considered obvious.

Commercial Surrogacy

The differences between the two decisions have helped set the parameters for the debate over the ethics of commercial surrogacy. The argument in favor of allowing payment of a fee to surrogates beyond their reasonable expenses has taken one of two forms. First, it is argued that commercial surrogacy is essentially not equivalent to baby selling. Instead, the fee is payment for gestational services rendered. Second, it is granted that surrogacy does constitute baby selling, but the argument is made on the grounds that surrogacy is qualitatively different from the types of situations that the baby selling laws were designed to prevent. This viewpoint will argue that commercial surrogacy is indeed the sale of children, and that the differences between surrogacy and black market adoptions do not justify allowing for payment of a fee to surrogates. Thus, commercial surrogacy should be prohibited, and consideration paid to surrogates should only be for necessary medical expenses and other expenses associated with the pregnancy.

Twenty-five states currently have laws that prohibit the exchange of consideration for adoption of a child. These laws were enacted to prevent economically and emotionally vulnerable birth mothers from being coerced into giving up children for adoption that under non-coercive circumstances they would not otherwise give up. The abuses and excesses of black market adoptions were, and still are, the target of these laws. As applied to surrogacy, however, these

1. In the 1988 *Baby M* case, surrogate mother Mary Beth Whitehead was recognized as the legal mother of the child she carried as part of a surrogacy contract.

laws have been interpreted by the courts in different ways. For example, in Michigan and New Jersey, the laws have been applied to prohibit any commercialization of surrogacy. But in Kentucky, the courts have ruled that surrogacy does not fall under the heading of baby selling because the natural father cannot buy back what is already his. Kentucky's interpretation of adoption statutes seems to be the exception rather than the rule, since the surrogacy laws in the states that have enacted them are generally consistent with existing adoption laws.

An Argument for Commercial Surrogacy

The Fee Is for Services Rendered, Not for the Sale of a Child. Though this argument takes various forms, proponents insist that surrogacy is not inherently baby selling, since the fee that is paid to the surrogate is for her gestational services, and thus constitutes simply another expense for the contracting couple, parallel to the medical and legal expenses involved. This argument assumes sensitivity to existing adoption laws, being careful to delineate exactly the things for which the fee pays, and insuring that the transfer of parental rights is not included under that heading. Most surrogacy contracts are structured to relate the fee to the specific gestational services rendered by the surrogate, and those who frame the contracts are careful not to make any mention of surrendering parental rights as part of the services for which the fee is paid.

Among the various forms that this argument can take, William Laufer suggests that the contracting couple does not buy the child, but rather buys the woman's egg and rents her womb, emphatically denying that the couple pays for an adoption. Avi Katz suggests that the fee pays for the entire process, not just the final step in it, and thus calls surrogacy contracts to bear a child, not contracts to sell a child. Karen Marie Sly terms surrogacy not baby selling, but prenatal baby-sitting, and the surrogate has the right to rent her womb for a fee. This definition of surrogacy is the foundation for her argument that prohibiting commercial surrogacy violates a woman's constitutional right to contract. Lori Andrews draws a parallel between the fee paid to surrogates and the other payments to those involved in helping relieve infertility. She states, "Prohibiting payment to the surrogate is as much an interference with the couple's reproductive rights as passing a law which bans payment to doctors who perform in vitro fertilization or a law which bans payment to pharmacists for contraceptives."

She parallels that analogy with an analogy drawn between childrearing and childbearing. It is legitimate to pay for all kinds of services involved in childrearing, from wet nurses to day care. Since childrearing, not childbearing, is the more influential element in the child's well being in the long run, if it is justifiable to pay people for childrearing, then surely it is valid to pay them for childbearing. Finally, Christine Sistare insists that all the attention being paid to baby selling is a "red herring" that distracts from the real issue of a woman's autonomy and a male fear that women's reproductive capacities will no longer be available cheaply or on demand.

The Intended End of Surrogacy

The argument that the surrogacy fee is for services and not for the sale of a child fails to take into account both the nature of the surrogacy contract and the intended end of a surrogacy arrangement. Most surrogacy contracts are structured around the product, not the process or the service of surrogacy. For example, the Stern-Whitehead contract specified that only in the event that Mary Beth Whitehead delivered a healthy baby to the Sterns would she be paid the entire $10,000 fee. If she miscarried prior to the fifth month of pregnancy, she would receive no fee, though all medical expenses would be paid. If she miscarried after the fifth month, or if the child was stillborn, she would only receive $1,000 of the fee. The contract was oriented to delivery of the end product, not the service rendered in the process. Normally, the majority of the fee (usually half), if not all of it (as was the case with the Stern-Whitehead case), is withheld until parental rights are actually waived and the custody of the child is turned over to the contracting couple. Thus, it is difficult to see how the fee can be for gestational services only when the service itself is not the final intent of the contract. Payment is made upon the surrogate fulfilling all the necessary responsibilities to insure the transfer of parental rights. Alexander M. Capron and Margaret J. Radin of the University of Southern California Law Center suggest that the claim that the fee is for gestational services alone is merely a disguise that serves to hide the true intent of the contract. They state, "The claim that the payment to the surrogate is merely for 'gestational services' is just a pretense, since payment is made 'upon surrender of custody' of the child and for 'carrying out obligations' under the agreement. These include taking all steps necessary to establish the biological father's paternity and to transfer all parental rights to the biological father and his mate.". . .

Baby Selling

Commercial surrogacy is indeed baby selling and should be prohibited. Given the long tradition in the United States against the sale of human beings, as with slavery and with children through adoption laws, the burden is on the advocates of commercial surrogacy to show either that it does not involve the sale of children or that it is an acceptable form of it. Most of the arguments in favor of commercial surrogacy are sensitive to the charge of baby selling, and supporters go to considerable lengths to show that it is not, or that if it is, it is benign in its effects. . . .

There is not much controversy in American society concerning the morality of selling children. Most agree that children should not be objects of barter, both for utilitarian and deontological reasons. The real debate in surrogacy is whether the practice does indeed constitute the sale of children, and if it does, whether this makes a morally significant difference. The conclusion of this viewpoint is that surrogacy is the equivalent of selling children, and does not constitute an acceptable form of baby selling.

The first argument made by proponents of commercial surrogacy is that the fee paid to the surrogate is payment for gestational services, not for the sale of a child. Yet upon closer examination, a substantial portion of the fee pays for the willingness of the surrogate to waive parental rights to the child she is carrying. Many surrogacy contracts include provisions that the balance of the fee, if not all of it, will be held in escrow until the arrangement is completed, that is, until the child is turned over to the contracting couple and adopted by the natural father's wife. These contracts also often include provisions that the surrogate will receive less of the fee should she miscarry or give birth to a stillborn child. The contract and payment schedule are oriented to the product of the arrangement, not to the process. If it were process oriented, the surrogate would receive the same fee whether she turned over the child or not, a situation inconceivable to surrogacy brokers. Thus, the way the fee is paid indicates that it is indeed for the waiver of parental rights, precisely the thing that adoption laws were written to preclude, since such a waiver for a fee constitutes baby selling.

Black Market Adoptions

A second argument attempts to distance surrogacy from the practice that the adoption laws were written to discourage, black market adoptions. Proponents suggest that there are major differences between the two practices. . . . The differences were either overstated or not relevant to the discussion of surrogacy. For example, one major difference is that the adopting father is the child's natural father, as opposed to a stranger. However, genetics alone does not necessarily make for a better parent, and simply because the natural father is involved in the transaction does not make it any less of a transaction. He is not the sole owner of the child, but a joint tenant with the surrogate. He is, in effect, buying out the surrogate's rights to the child with the fee. A further difference is that surrogacy is concerned with the child's best interests as opposed to black market adoptions which are solely financially driven. Yet this overstates the difference, since the only psychological screening done in surrogacy is on the surrogate, and normally the only screening done on the contracting couple is financial. A third difference is that in surrogacy, coercion of the surrogate cannot take place since the agreement is entered into prior to the onset of pregnancy. Thus there is no unwanted pregnancy that might coerce a young unwed mother, for example, to give her child up when she would not do so under less coercive circumstances. But to suggest that surrogacy is free from coercion overstates the case, since once the pregnancy begins and the surrogate decides she wants to keep the child, she may have a wanted pregnancy and an unwanted contract that will force her to give up the child she is carrying.

Reproductive Freedom

Philosopher Thomas Hurka argued that if women have the right to abortion, then other reproductive practices such as surrogate motherhood might be granted on the same grounds that women have the right to decide about their own reproductive activities. What is being overlooked here is the ethical distinction between a woman's being forced by an outside agency to carry an unwanted pregnancy to term, and the deliberate action of becoming pregnant for the purpose of selling a child to others.

One cannot equate women's right to access to abortion with a "right" to conceive and give birth to children for the purpose of selling them, without doing violence to basic ethical reasoning. Reproductive freedom is about the ordering, or cultivation of unconscious, natural processes by conscious human agents. Men have always reserved the right to act upon nature; why should women not have a similar right to act upon their own individual natural processes in the context of directing their own lives?

Marsha Hewitt, *Canadian Dimension*, September 1991.

A third argument attempts to draw a parallel between AID [artificial insemination by donor] and surrogacy. Proponents of commercial surrogacy insist that since AID is legitimate, and men can be paid a nominal amount for sperm donation, women should also be able to engage in surrogacy for a fee. But the more appropriate parallel to AID is not surrogacy, but egg donation. Equal protection only requires that women be able to donate their eggs for a small fee in the same way that men donate their sperm. . . .

Violence to Children's Personhood

Further arguments include the fact that children are not treated as commodities in surrogacy and that money changes hands in some adoption proceedings. It is true that the majority of children born to surrogates are well treated by their new families. But the fact remains that they are still being bought and sold. Even though there were certainly slaves who were treated well, that hardly justifies the sale of human beings. In response to the concept of money changing hands in some adoption proceedings, the permitted exchange of money in adoption occurs between two already existing parents, not between two people who have been strangers prior to the surrogacy arrangement being organized. Further, the exchange of cash, as in surrogacy, has been banned even between already existing family members. The consideration being exchanged in the cases being used to support this argument was forgiveness of a debt or a child support obligation, not a cash deal as is the case in surrogacy.

The most obvious argument against commercial surrogacy is that it constitutes the sale of children, violating adoption laws in many states as well as the Thirteenth Amendment. Commercial surrogacy is prohibited because it involves the commodification of children, that is, it is one of the blocked exchanges, blocked because of society's desire to protect certain areas of social life from the realm of the market. Baby selling is blocked because babies are market inalienable, that is, because human beings cannot be bought and sold without doing violence to an essential aspect of personhood.

Exploitation of the Surrogate

Further arguments against commercial surrogacy include the notions that women's reproductive capacities should not be subject to the dictates of the market. However, it is not clear that surrogacy involves a morally objectionable market transaction: only the sale of the child that results from the agreement is inherently morally objectionable. What makes the commodification of women's reproductive services argument more compelling is the potential for exploitation of the surrogate. Although such exploitation has not materialized so far, there is evidence of surrogacy brokers marketing surrogacy among poor women, particularly those in the Third World, and thus the potential for exploiting women is real.

The main objection to commercial surrogacy is that it is the equivalent of baby selling, a practice that is inherently morally objectionable, because human beings are not objects of barter or commerce. Any attempt to show that surrogacy does not constitute child selling fails to account for the realities of the surrogacy contract. Thus, public policy should be formulated to prohibit a fee to surrogates beyond reasonable medical expenses and perhaps lost wages due to the pregnancy. Any fee to surrogacy brokers to set up a commercial surrogacy arrangement should likewise be prohibited.

"The opposition to postmenopausal pregnancies . . . 'expresses a prejudice against what is new or unconventional, rather than a position that can be rationally justified.'"

Postmenopausal Pregnancies Should Be Permitted

Lawrence M. Hinman

Lawrence M. Hinman is a professor of philosophy and ethics at the University of San Diego and author of *Contemporary Moral Issues: Diversity and Consensus*. In the following viewpoint, Hinman contends that the opposition to postmenopausal pregnancies cannot be justified on the basis of age. He contests the argument that it is in the best interest of the child not to have older parents because they have limited parenting capabilities. On the contrary, Hinman suggests that older parents may have advantages over young parents, including financial security and the emotional maturity that comes with personal experience.

As you read, consider the following questions:

1. How does Hinman counter the view that the likelihood of older parents to die earlier than younger parents threatens the best interest of the child?
2. According to the author, how is restricting older parents' reproductive options similar to restricting the reproductive options of the disabled?
3. In the author's opinion, what is one reason why a person or couple may want to have children later in life?

S hortly after a fifty-nine year old British woman, Jennifer
F., gave birth to twins at Dr. Severino Antinori's fertility
clinic in Rome and—six months later—Rosanna Della Corte
gave birth at the age of 62 to a baby boy at the same clinic,
the French government introduced a bill to prohibit postmenopausal pregnancies. The French Health Minister, Dr.
Philippe Douste-Blazy, argued that "artificial late pregnancies were immoral as well as dangerous to the health of
mother and child . . . [and] urged women not to be 'egoistic'
by trying to become pregnant after menopause." Dr. John
Marks, former chairman of the British Medical Association
Council, said the woman's case "bordered on the Franken-
stein syndrome." Virginia Bottomley, Britain's secretary of
state for health, said, "Women do not have the right to have
a child; the child has a right to a suitable home." Similar restrictions were introduced in the Italian legislature in the
wake of a papal encyclical, *Evangelium Vitae*, condemning in
vitro fertilization and many other high-tech fertility procedures. Italy's Association of Medical Practitioners and Den-
tists barred their members from administering fertility treatment to women over fifty. Italy's National Council of the
Federation of Doctors barred artificial inseminations for all
but child-bearing age heterosexual married couples. Indeed,
this and other similar cases have given rise to considerable
controversy about what the contours of procreative liberty
ought to be in regard to age. . . .

The Opposition to Older Parents

The opposition to older parents seems to stem from several
sources. The opposition to postmenopausal pregnancies, as
Bonnie Steinbock and Ron McClamrock have pointed out in
a 1994 article in *The Hastings Center Report*, probably "expresses a prejudice against what is new or unconventional,
rather than a position that can be rationally justified." . . .
The opposition is, in this country I suspect, also a symptom
of a youth culture that values youth and energy over age and
experience. In some countries where life expectancy is low, it
may also stem from an understandable experience of the local life span of parents.

The interesting philosophical issue here is whether such

age restrictions on parenting have a *rational* foundation. Several arguments can be advanced in support of such restrictions. All of these arguments appeal in some way to the best interests of the child. Each has some merit, and each points to a genuine moral concern. However, none of these arguments is sufficient to establish a strong restriction on age per se, and indeed, none of these arguments proves to be genuinely age-based. Each of these arguments points to factors that, while associated with age, are not tied to it in a direct and univocal way. Let's examine each of these arguments.

The Best Interests of the Child Arguments

One of the most common arguments against postmenopausal pregnancies . . . is that they are unfair to the child, that they harm the children in some way. Indeed, there is widespread agreement in . . . the world of *in vitro* fertilization . . . that the welfare of the child should be the principal—perhaps the sole—concern in making these decisions. It is not in the best interest of the child, this argument implies, to have older parents. . . .

What are the harms that we are talking about here? Presumably these are harms that result from the age of the parents, especially of the mother. (I'll consider the issue of gender equity below.) The case against older parents has two aspects: the age of the parent's death relative to the age of the child, and the parent's age and associated energy level relative to the child's. Let's consider each of these.

The Death of the Parent. The thrust of this objection is that older parents are more likely than parents who are younger to die when their children are still young. In the British case of the woman who had twins at the age of fifty-nine, she is much more likely to die while the children are still growing up than if she had had children when she was in her twenties or thirties.

Yet for this argument to be sound, it would have to include more cases than just postmenopausal women. The underlying principle is presumably something like this:

> Individuals should not have children when there is a higher than normal chance that they will die before the children have reached adulthood.

There are several difficulties with this principle.

First, it makes a major life decision dependent on a highly fallible judgment. Our ability to predict life span in any individual case is far from reliable, and we may well be ill advised to place so much weight on such a judgment. The weightier the decision, the more we justifiably expect certitude.

Second, this principle would be more restrictive than most of us would like. It would limit not only people with a potentially lethal disease, but also anyone who has an above average susceptibility to such diseases. At a time in our history when we are trying to affirm the rights of persons with disabilities of various kinds, a principle such as this one threatens to restrict persons with disabilities in one of the most important areas of human life. This concern is further exacerbated by continuing developments in genetic screening and our consequent ability to foresee possible illnesses.

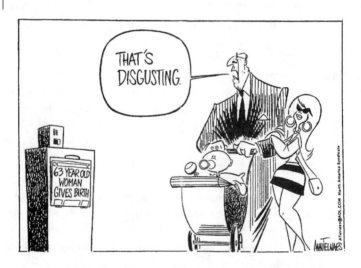

Telnaes. © 1997 by North American Syndicate. Reprinted with permission.

Third, it treats the death of a parent as a supreme evil. Yet the issue is more complex. The harm of the death of a parent is certainly a sad and sometimes even tragic event, but the harm associated with it has to be seen in conjunction with the goods attendant upon having had that particular person as a parent. All of this . . . has to be balanced against the possible goods and harms associated with (in the post-menopausal pregnancy case) not having been born at all. . . .

Finally, we can legitimately question whether the only interest that counts in this equation is the interest of the child. . . . Such decisions should be guided, it is implied, solely by a consideration for the best interests of the child. The implication is that other interests do not count. . . .

In what ways, if any, should the interests of potential parents enter into this equation? It seems reasonable that they should in principle be given at least some weight. We will return to this issue below, when we consider motives for post-menopausal pregnancies . . . later in life.

The Parenting Capabilities Argument

The second principal concern that gives rise to age restrictions relates to the physical capabilities of the parents. Because of their age, this argument states, older parents will be less able to do many of the things that contribute to the well-being of the child than younger parents can do.

What are these things? Typically, proponents of this argument point to physical activities such as playing baseball and soccer with children. The person who becomes a parent at fifty-nine will begin playing soccer with his or her children in the early to mid-sixties. Most of us peak well before this age in terms of our athletic abilities. Advocates of these age restrictions may also point to social limitations. It is difficult for the child, they maintain, when the child's parents are the only ones at a child's school gathering with gray, or perhaps even white, hair. Finally, some advocates of age restrictions may even maintain that older parents, on the whole, are less physically energetic than their younger counterparts. Therefore, such parents have less energy for their children.

One of the difficulties with this argument is that it goes too far in its restrictions. Think of the cases which such a restriction might cover.

- *The Bookworm Case.* If physical capabilities, especially in areas such as sports, are required for parenthood, many of us who are not so inclined or gifted might well be restricted from becoming parents.

- *Persons with Disabilities.* Similar issues arise in regard to persons with disabilities, whether these be purely physical or are also social. Should someone in a wheelchair be refused the opportunity for parenthood solely on the basis of that condition?
- *The Prematurely Gray.* Finally, there are people who simply look much older than they actually are. Sometimes this is due to premature grayness of the hair, sometimes to premature wrinkles, etc.

Thus we begin to see that these attempts to restrict parenthood on the basis of age fall short of the mark. They fail to establish that age necessarily entails characteristics detrimental to the best interests of the child; furthermore, they fail to show that only age is associated with those characteristics. Finally, they fail to show that those characteristics are necessarily detrimental to the best interests of the child. . . .

The other question to ask here is whether older parents bring to parenting any special characteristics not usually found in younger parents.

Generalizations about the differences between older and younger parents are notoriously difficult, and any claims about them are best couched in hypothetical terms. That said, we can see some possible advantages. Older parents are more likely to be financially secure than their younger counterparts. Second, they are more likely to be under less pressure in their chosen profession than those who are just beginning and must continually prove themselves. Presumably this means that they will be more able, all other things being equal, to have disposable time that they can spend with their children. Finally, many older parents would claim that they have much more emotional maturity than they had twenty or even ten years earlier. That emotional maturity, they claim, allows them to raise their children in a more sensitive manner than they would otherwise be able to do.

The Gender-Bias Argument

There is obviously another major argument against restricting postmenopausal pregnancies: these restrictions fall solely on women. They do not limit men in the same way, at least in part because it is difficult to regulate or limit the reproductive activities of men. Yet it is simply a fact of nature that women, once they have gone through menopause, cannot conceive without technological assistance. Men, even in advanced age, can father children without necessarily needing technological assistance. Thus women are more vulnerable to controls on their reproductive freedoms than men are. I would certainly want to reject any proposed restriction that singled out women alone in this fashion.

It is striking, in this context, to look at the newspaper reports of the birth of Rosanna Della Corte's son Ricardo. Great outrage was expressed over the fact that she was sixty-two; hardly a mention was made over the fact that her husband was in his sixties.

Indeed, it is helpful in this context to see the issue of age restrictions . . . postmenopausal pregnancies . . . as a choice issue. Defenders of reproductive freedom have long emphasized a woman's right *not* to have a child, but the other side of a pro-choice position is presumably the right *to* have a child. Opposing age restrictions is, I think, part of being pro-choice. . . .

Wise Choices

To argue that individuals should have the maximal degree of liberty in making reproductive choices obviously does not mean that all such choices are wise ones. Let me conclude with several remarks on what we could call the contours of reproductive wisdom.

The Motivation Issue. Stories of postmenopausal pregnancy are often greeted with incredulity about why someone would want to have a child (much less twins) at such a late time in life. Why do older persons have, or want to have, children beyond the usual childbearing age?

The answers to this question are, in large measure, the same answers we find in parents of a younger age. The relevant question is perhaps why they didn't act on those reasons earlier in their life. As we shall see, in at least some of these cases, they did act on those reasons earlier in life.

We can imagine several common scenarios. First, a child might have died, and the person might want to have another child in its place, as it were. There are certainly serious dangers with any attempt to have one child "replace" another, but there is nothing about these dangers that is confined to older age. This indeed was the principal motivation in the case of Rosanna Della Corte, whose sixteen year old son Ricardo had died in an automobile accident three years earlier. The baby she had at sixty-two was also named Ricardo.

Second, a woman might have been infertile—either all her life or during the period when she wanted to have children—and only with the development of new technologies is she at last able to conceive. Her reasons for having children may be no different than anyone else's. However, the technology necessary to allow her to conceive may have only been developed when she was postmenopausal.

Third, we can imagine a person wanting to have children with a new spouse after getting married later in life. (This in fact has been the motivation in several cases.) This seems to be a thoroughly reasonable motivation. There may be a variety of factors that make it an unwise choice, and the likelihood of these factors may increase with age, but it hardly seems that age alone should be an impediment here.

Preserving the Option

The Seasons of Life Issue. A final argument here is worthy of consideration, although it is hard to state it with precision. Isn't it the case that life has, as it were, its seasons and that having children late in life—whether for males or females—is to ignore those seasons?

There is, I think, merit in this argument, but it is hardly strong enough to justify restriction on having children later in life. The seasons certainly are there, but it is also true that we live increasingly in an age of choice, one where we may construct lives that do not follow traditional patterns. It is important, I think, to continue to preserve this as an option.

> "*Postmenopausal [pregnancy] is more likely to oppress than to 'rescue' or provide equity for women.*"

Postmenopausal Pregnancies Should Be Banned

Abby Lippman

In the following viewpoint, Abby Lippman claims that reproductive technologies should not be used to give post-menopausal women the option of pregnancy. Lippman argues these reproductive technologies impose sexist expectations upon women to assume the roles of childbearers and mothers. She contends that menopause is a natural part of womanhood, not a biological shortcoming or a health problem. Lippman is a professor of epidemiology and biostatistics at McGill University in Montreal, Canada.

As you read, consider the following questions:

1. According to the author, between what ages does menopause occur for healthy North American women?
2. How does Lippman support her claim that reproductive technology puts pressure on menopausal women to become pregnant?
3. In Lippman's opinion, how does menopause provide relief for women?

Excerpted from "Never Too Late: Biotechnology, Women, and Reproduction," by Abby Lippman, *McGill Law Journal* (New York: McGraw-Hill, 1995). Copyright © 1995 by McGraw-Hill, Inc. Reprinted with permission.

"**B**iotechnology, women and reproduction": the phrase combines in one breath a dangerous trio. This viewpoint focuses on but one area where these words intersect and where the dangers to women emerge clearly: postmenopausal pregnancy. This area is representative of many others where reproductive technology claims to have "rescued" women by offering us body management, control and choice. In this case, the lauded "rescue" is said to be from age limitations on fertility; postmenopausal obstetrics, by managing our aging bodies, will now offer women not only pregnancy at any age but, in the process, "equity" with men.

In this viewpoint, I want to begin to uncover how postmenopausal obstetrics is more likely to oppress than to "rescue" or provide equity for women. Further, I want to suggest that this oppression results directly from the ideology of postmenopausal obstetrics that uses technology to adapt women to men's biographies and reinforces negative stereotypes of the aging female. . . .

Pregnancy After Menopause

The spontaneous cessation of ovulation and the resulting termination of reproductive capacity in women are what we generally label menopause. For the average healthy North American woman who has not been surgically sterilized, this process usually occurs sometime between the ages of forty-eight and fifty-one, with most women's experiences falling within a range of forty-five to fifty-five years of age. About 0.3 per cent of women under this age have non-surgically induced lack of ovaries or of ovulation, usually called ovarian "failure", so that, with respect to reproduction, they are functionally menopausal.

Biomedical researchers are now offering to create pregnancies for these women who have experienced menopause or are functionally menopausal. This is done through: the purchase of eggs from younger women; laboratory or *in vitro* fertilization (IVF) and transfer of a woman's eggs; and the hormonal manipulation of women carrying the fertilized eggs. For simplicity, I shall refer to all of these generically as postmenopausal pregnancies. . . .

I will put aside two of the most obvious problems with

postmenopausal pregnancy, namely how this is but one more manifestation of the previously well-described medicalization of women's health, and how the experimental procedures involved have an abysmal failure rate and pose considerable and serious risks to the woman and to the fetus. Instead, I will focus on how, despite the biomedical rhetoric of "liberating" women from their life cycles, the possibilities and practice of postmenopausal obstetrics are actually quite oppressive.

Oppression and Postmenopausal Pregnancy

I take as given that there is no such thing as "natural" old— or middle—age. All of us, women and men, age within a sociopolitical and cultural context that gives meaning to personal chronology. Stripped of its accompanying context, aging is but a decrease in the numerical probability of continuing to live. It is a universal *experience* of all living organisms. All who are born do age, with some merely involved in the process for longer than others.

But age is never isolated to this extent other than, perhaps, in actuarial tables from insurance companies. Rather, as with gender, race, ability and other "signifiers", it is a notion of difference that comes clothed in various socially constituted presumptions and attitudes. Moreover, in North America, because it is a difference that matters, age is both socially constituted and politically invented.

Oppression thus first emerges in the ageism and sexism of this technology. Postmenopausal pregnancy fits into the sexist and capitalist definition of women as producers of children: only because (certain) women are *expected* to be mothers regardless of age could the *inability* to be pregnant at, for example, forty-eight years or older, possibly be seen as "infertility". Assuming childbearing is a necessary and sufficient source of fulfilment for the older woman, postmenopausal pregnancy perpetuates the ageist image of the woman in middle and older age who is no longer productive by offering to "treat" this condition.

Postmenopausal pregnancy is also oppressive because it inverts—and otherwise plays with—notions of choice. If nothing else, women cannot "choose" to become pregnant after age fifty so much as physicians can choose (along the usual lines of discrimination such as class, ability, sexual orientation, *etc.*) those to whom to offer this technology. More troubling, however, is how *not* being pregnant after menopause can no longer be seen, because of the technological advances, as an inevitable stage in a biological cycle; rather, it too has become a "choice".

The Pressure to Conform

Granted, for some women this "choice" to become pregnant after menopause, to carry out women's traditional role in a conventional way, is an active *response* to societal sexism and ageism that has limited their other options for self-fulfilment and recognition and is not merely a passive submission to these forces. After all, we *do* embody social and cultural norms. Nevertheless, it remains the case that the mere availability of this technology means that a woman who does *not* undergo it can be presented as having "chosen" to forgo bearing a child, as having "chosen" not to do all she can for her partner who wants a child, as having "chosen" not to assume the womanly role expected of her or as having "chosen" not to control her biology.

The technology thereby puts additional pressure on women to conform to existing gendered norms. Those who might have found release from pressures to be pregnant with the welcome arrival of menopause now have an indeterminate sentence and become at risk for "victim-blaming"—it is now *her* fault if she is not pregnant. Who will have sympathy for one who has "chosen" not to control her body when she could? After all, surrounded by media-generated images that depict the aging woman in a battle with time, fighting against wrinkles or increased weight or her "biological clock", why would a financially comfortable white North American woman *not* want to enter combat and welcome the opportunity to become an alleged "winner"? With a cult of "eternal youth" generating additional pressures on us to control our bodies, it seems consistent for a woman to assent to "rescue" from her biology and release from its constraints—especially if other "escapes" from becoming devalued are foreclosed. Thus, it might be more appropriate to see having, or not having, a postmenopausal pregnancy as an individual, yet socially conditioned *action*. However, as a response to a social context that promotes this activity, it is not necessarily an individual choice.

Further, we might ask if it is liberating to circumvent a process that has been among those defining us as women, for the chance to "succeed" on men's terms. Is it liberating to be "rescued" from women's biology so as to be situated, for purposes of fertility, in men's biology and thus to be re-housed in the male-defined institute called "family", with this transfer camouflaged by the language of choice? . . .

Distinctions Between Childlessness and Infertility

Oppression also results because postmenopausal pregnancies blur important distinctions between childlessness, a social situation remedied simply by the presence of a child, and "infertility", the medical condition of a woman who is physiologically or anatomically unable to conceive. This conceptual confusion again perpetuates the institutionalized idea of a family based on male definitions. This oppression extends to all women because it distracts us from adopting the necessary measures to prevent infertility and to provide social support for childlessness. If one can take eggs from a woman when she is young and freeze them for her or another woman's later use, we should question whether there would be any impetus to remove those workplace hazards that jeopardize fertility and themselves create the window of opportunity for high-tech "rescues". Here, as elsewhere when new genetic and reproductive technologies are involved, what seem to be "private" decisions actually affect us all and can easily result in public consequences, if not in collective harm. Even if the public and private realms were not socio-cultural constructs with a constantly changing frontier, all of us would be affected by the development and use of these interventions. . . .

Biomedical—and some media—enthusiasm for post-menopausal pregnancies rests primarily on the implicit assumption that if women, like men, can indefinitely retain their biological capacity to produce a child, the equity between the sexes, now impossible because women's physiology is a "natural" barrier to it, will be fostered:

When men have children in their old age, it's looked on as a kind of crowning achievement in their lives . . . To say that simply because these women are postmenopausal and above the age of 50 they can't provide adequate child care to a baby, that is patently ridiculous [Dr. Mark Siegler, *The New York Times*, January 2, 1994].

Another assumption is that menopause is always and necessarily unwelcome although many women may, in fact, look forward to the relief it provides from such things as menstrual symptoms, worry about accidental pregnancies, and, for those who have for many years been unable or unwilling to become pregnant, from prying questions about why they are not yet pregnant. Freedom from the ability to become pregnant may be, for some, even more valuable than being "free" to become pregnant at any age.

The Beginning of Positive Changes

"We often hear about the negative impacts of growing older or reaching menopause," said Wulf Utian, M.D., the executive director of the North American Menopause Society (NAMS), "yet when we ask women, we continually hear that they view menopause as the beginning of many positive changes in their lives and health." Among the positive changes, women included improvement in family or home life, sense of personal fulfillment, ability to focus on hobbies and other interests, relationship with spouse or partner, and friendships.

Menopause News, September 1998.

As postmenopausal obstetrics emerges, it is being promoted as a humane response to the needs of women who "chose" to postpone childbearing while they pursued education and careers. Unfortunately, this view completely ignores how only *some* women may have the luxury to complete their educations or to establish their careers and to postpone pregnancy. It overlooks how postmenopausal obstetrics is but another franchise of the "business that caters to those who will make a business out of being a family" [as stated by M. Strathern]. In this business, women's eggs are a kind of "therapeutic" merchandise and children become luxury items to be purchased from the best suppliers, with women's bodies the "cultural plastic" [in the words of S. Bordo] out of which they are fashioned. This industry ignores how postponing or delaying pregnancy is not necessarily a real choice when the privileged white man's traditional unbroken, linear career path is imposed as the norm to which women are expected to adapt. To the extent that "delay" is constructed by societal norms, postmenopausal pregnancy only offers to "resolve" what should not have even been a problem. . . .

Biopolitical, Not Biomedical

Technology is never neutral; when applied to women it is necessarily gendered in ways that reflect and support prevailing attitudes and customs. Postmenopausal pregnancy mirrors and reinforces the "production of baby" metaphor that dominates much of the recent biomedical literature about pregnancy. It is advanced as a tool to reverse, or to "rescue" us from, age-based cessation of egg production—in essence, to rejuvenate us. It partakes of a view of female aging as a disease-causing agent, a view with great potential to constrain needed social changes.

There is nothing obviously "natural" about age. Age in a broader sense, however, is a complex socially defined construct: cultural, social and political contexts influence how and when we age. Some of this complexity is revealed in the way we generally assume the existence of such things as chronological age, mental age and social ages (for example, driving-age, voting-age, drinking-age, retirement-age, golden-age). Yet, it is important to remember that all these are tied to what society allows us to do as well as to available technologies. As such, ages are flexible, with boundaries that vary according to political decisions, technological developments and so on. Childbearing-age has joined this list as a category that rests on biopolitical, perhaps even more than on biomedical decisions.

Postmenopausal pregnancy is a costly way—financially, physically and emotionally—for women to conform to male biography. Oppression is more likely than liberation to result from its practice. We must learn to value the older woman and *her own* trajectory. This requires us to remove the real constraints to graceful aging for most women, those that stem from poverty, abuse and discriminatory social and economic policies that damage our health. The problems experienced by aging women are not created by the fact of living many years, but they do result from the lack of resources and the abuse and denigration that await us. Privileging postmenopausal pregnancy and other cosmetic fixes is more likely to exacerbate women's aging-related problems. If we instead focused on these broader social problems, we might begin to reclaim our right to define ourselves on our own terms and reject the male biomedical model on which the marketing of postmenopausal pregnancy is based.

When I stop releasing eggs, it will not be because I have "failed" biologically; rather, I will have reached a perfectly expected, albeit new, stage in my life. At this stage, I want to be free to act my age, both unconstrained and not passing as someone else. It should be liberating to accept this new limit on my body and, perhaps, even see it as an advantage. Did I really enjoy menstrual cramps? Invariably searching for a tampon in unfriendly places? Has not menopause itself actually "rescued" me from these? I might even enjoy this stage if policies and their accompanying interventions eliminate poverty, abuse and isolation, and provide safety, security, value and equity—rather than pregnancy—to women fifty years and older.

Feminists have generally been critical of environmentally unfriendly behaviour towards women. We recognize threats to our health as resulting from the ideologies of patriarchy, capitalism and technological reductionism. In our response to these most recent technologies, which are imbued with the same ideologies, we must keep these threats in mind.

Not About Disability, Deficiency or Disease

Menopause is not about disability, deficiency or disease. Why not reimagine this rhythm in the lives of women and refuse attempts to pass over the aging process (if for no other reason than it is probably too hard to do)? Do I really want to lop off old(er) age as if it were a bothersome skinfold? Do I want to be seen as [in the words of M. Lock] a "perambulatory anomaly"? Shall I be a "lavendar rose" or a "grey panther"; a senior citizen or a Raging Grannie? Do I want to guard an empty nest, re-stock it with fledgling dillings or fly the coop? If I become a "Methusaleh mom" following a "retirement pregnancy" will I not be cheated of the wonderful things my age should allow me to do? When I am too old to work, should I not also be too old to work at staying young, as biomedicine would encourage me to do?

Perhaps there are some things which we, as individuals and as a society, are better off accepting and yielding to than struggling against or seeking to fix through biomedicine and reproductive technologies. Age seems to be one experience we might consider in this light.

Periodical Bibliography

The following articles have been selected to supplement the diverse views presented in this chapter. Addresses are provided for periodicals not indexed in the *Readers' Guide to Periodical Literature*, the *Alternative Press Index*, the *Social Sciences Index*, or the *Index to Legal Periodicals and Books*.

Lori B. Andrews	"No More Custom-Made Babies," *Self*, April 2000.
Carl Djerassi	"Sex in an Age of Mechanical Reproduction," *Science*, July 2, 1999.
Julia Duin	"Reckless Reproduction?" *Insight on the News*, July 19, 1999.
Ezekiel J. Emanuel	"The Case Against Octuplets: Eight Is Too Many," *New Republic*, January 25, 1999.
Anne Taylor Fleming	"Why I Can't Use Someone Else's Eggs: Are Women Fully Prepared for the Moral and Emotional Repercussions of Donor Eggs?" *Newsweek*, April 12, 1999.
Vida Foubister	"Reproductive Technologies Outpacing Ethical Consideration," *American Medical News*, January 17, 2000.
John Geddes, Susan McClelland, and Patricia Chisholm	"Making Babies: In the Age or In Vitro Fertilization, Does the State Have a Place in the Test Tubes of the Nation?" *Maclean's*, December 6, 1999.
Carey Goldberg	"Just Another Girl, Unlike Any Other," *New York Times*, October 27, 1999.
Phillip Hilts	"Largest Study Yet Rates Fertility Drugs," *New York Times*, January 21, 1999.
Claudia Kalb	"Families: The Octuplet Question," *Newsweek*, January 11, 1999.
Lance Morrow	"Is This Right? Who Has the Right to Say?" *Time*, January 11, 1999.
National Catholic Reporter	"In Vitro Fertilization Widely Used," October 22, 1999.
Elizabeth Pyton	"Is Surrogate Motherhood Moral?" *Humanist*, September 2001.
Alissa J. Ruben and Aaron Zitner	"Fertility Cases Spur an Illicit Drug Market," *Los Angeles Times*, September 10, 2000.
Washington Post	"Embryo Ethics," August 12, 2001.

CHAPTER 4

What Ethics Should Guide Genetic Research?

Chapter Preface

Many commentators claim that genetic research will greatly transform medicine. For example, genetic tests will allow doctors to determine an individual's likelihood to develop certain genetically based diseases. In addition, genetic manipulation may enable physicians to protect an embryo from the harmful effects of irregular genes. While debate surrounds such therapeutic uses of genetic science, the prospect of using genetic research for nontherapeutic uses—particularly in allowing parents to select or enhance their unborn child's physical or mental characteristics—is especially steeped in controversy.

Proponents argue that parents should be free to use genetic engineering to improve or choose their children's characteristics. According to one anonymous commentator, "Even before conception we 'naturally' intervene in how we want our offspring by choosing people we are attracted to for brains, looks, personality. . . . What's wrong with ensuring the best for your child at any stage of that child's development?" Others stress that parents reserve the right to build their families in ways they see fit. For instance, philosophy professor Gregory Pence asks, "Would it be so terrible to allow parents to at least aim for a certain type, in the same way that great breeders . . . try to match a breed of dogs to the needs of a family?"

However, opponents contend that allowing parents to genetically enhance or control the traits of their children would have negative social consequences. Some caution that genetic enhancement may be used to weed out certain human traits. For example, author Cathy Young insists that some people may want to "provide early reparative therapy to embryos carrying the gay gene" in order to do away with homosexuality. Furthermore, others assert that genetic enhancement will only be accessible to the privileged and will further polarize social classes. Law professor Patricia J. Williams alleges that genetic engineering would offer affluent parents "racial and class superiority in a designer bottle."

In the following chapter, authors deliberate over what ethics should guide genetic research and the social and moral implications of genetic engineering.

"Genetics in particular will be fundamental to many science and technology areas and societal functions, including health and medicine."

Genetic Engineering Could Benefit Society

Joseph F. Coates, John B. Mahaffie, and Andy Hines

In the following viewpoint, Joseph F. Coates, John B. Mahaffie, and Andy Hines contend that genetic engineering promises to vastly improve life in the twenty-first century. The authors assert that genetic technologies could enable humans to detect and eliminate numerous genetic diseases and disorders, beneficially redirecting the course of evolution. Furthermore, they claim that plants and livestock could be genetically manipulated to enhance human health and the environment. Coates, Mahaffie, and Hines are authors of *2025: Scenarios of U.S. and Global Society Reshaped by Science and Technology*, on which this viewpoint is based.

As you read, consider the following questions:
1. According to Coates, Mahaffie, and Hines, how does genetics benefit forensics today?
2. In the authors' view, in what ways will genetic engineering allow farmers to improve their livestock?
3. Why do the authors state that genetic engineering will not be a "panacea" for all human ailments?

The twenty-first century may prove to be the Age of the Gene. Biotechnology promises dramatic improvements in agriculture, health care, manufacturing, and even human beings themselves.

Genetics will be a key enabling technology of the twenty-first century, rivaling information technology, materials technology, and energy technology in importance.

The effects of all of these enabling technologies will be far-reaching across business and society, but advances in genetics in particular will be fundamental to many science and technology areas and societal functions, including health and medicine, food and agriculture, nanotechnology, and manufacturing.

One benefit of genetics that is already highly visible is in forensics. DNA identification will significantly enhance criminology. It may contribute to declines in violent crime, the identification of deadbeat parents, and the prevention of fraud. It may even deter rape and murder, as potential perpetrators fear leaving their DNA "fingerprints" on the scene.

Rising public interest in genetics is tied to the growing realization that humanity is capable of directly shaping its own and other species' evolution. We will no longer have to wait for nature's relatively slow natural selection. Genetics will bring the capability of speeding and redirecting evolution along paths of our choice. Eliminating genetic diseases, for instance, might take centuries through natural selection but could be accomplished in decades through genetic manipulation.

This power will doubtless inspire a profound global debate about how genetics should and should not be used.

The Genetic Economy

On the economic front, genetics could reward those who invest in it for the long haul. It is an industry for patient capital. Its spread over many industries will make it an increasingly important factor in the global economy.

Genetics is not a typical industry, in that it is not measured as a separate entity. It will be a part of, or embedded in, so many industries that government statisticians will not attempt such a measure. A good guess is that genetics will account for about 20% of gross domestic product, or roughly $2 trillion in 2025.

The early emphasis on using genetics to improve human health and battle disease will be supplemented with more exotic applications, such as manufacturing and materials, human enhancement, energy, environmental engineering, and species restoration and management. The food and agriculture industries, for example, are steadily expanding their use of genetics. Advances will come from applying what seem like isolated breakthroughs into a systems framework. For example, researchers working on eradicating a species of locust may develop a microorganism useful in converting crop wastes into biomass energy.

Genetics and Species Management

The genomes of many animals, fish, insects, and microorganisms will be worked out, leading to more refined management, control, and manipulation of their health and propagation—or their elimination.

• *Designer animals.* Routine genetic programs will be used to enhance animals used for food production, recreation, and even pets. Goats, for example, are especially well suited to genetic manipulation. In affluent nations, goats will be used for producing pharmaceutical compounds; in less-developed nations, goats will produce high-protein milk.

Livestock will be customized to increase growth, shorten gestation, and enhance nutritional value. Farmers will be able to order the genes they want from gene banks for transmission to local biofactories, where the animals with the desired characteristics will then be produced and shipped.

Transgenic animals, sharing the genes of two or more species, may be created to withstand rough environments. Genes from the hardy llama in South America, for example, could be introduced into camels in the Middle East—and vice versa—to greatly expand the range of each. Some species will be introduced into entirely new areas. Parrots may be modified to withstand cold North American temperatures, becoming a boon to bird watchers in the United States.

Transgenic pets may become popular: Genes from mild-mannered Labrador retrievers could be put into pit bull terrier genomes.

• *Pest control.* Genetics will play a central role in pest management. The arms race between insects and pesticides has been marked by humans winning battles, but insects winning the war. Genetics will turn the tide.

One method is to breed pheromones into surrounding plants to lure pests away from their intended prey. Pests will also be sterilized through genetic engineering to disrupt their populations. Genetically engineered resistance to pests will be common through such techniques as inducing the plants to produce their own protective or repellant compounds.

Insects that carry disease will also be targeted through genetic engineering to control their populations. It is hoped that malaria will soon be eliminated this way.

Plant Genetics

• *Boosting plants.* Future farmers may have near total control over plant genetics. Plants will give higher yields and be more resistant to disease, frost, drought, and stress. They will have higher protein, lower oil, and more efficient photosynthesis rates than ever before. Natural processes such as ripening will be enhanced and controlled.

Genetics will allow farmers to customize and fine-tune crops, building in flavor, sweeteners, and preservatives, while increasing nutritional value.

The first step in agrogenetics is to identify disease-resistant genes; the second step is to put them into plants. Eventually, plants will be genetically engineered to produce specific prevention factors against likely disease invaders.

Forestry will also benefit from genetics. Genetic manipulation will result in superior tree strains with disease resistance and improved productivity. Trees will be routinely engineered to allow nonchemical pulping for use in paper making. Genetic forests will also help in the global restoration of many denuded areas.

• *Engineering microorganisms.* Manufacturers will use engineered microorganisms to produce commodity and specialty chemicals, as well as medicines, vaccines, and drugs. Groups of microorganisms, often working in sequence as living factories, will produce useful compounds. They will also be widely used in agriculture, mining, resource upgrading, waste management, and environmental cleanup. Oil- and chemical-spill cleanups are a high-profile application.

The development of so-called suicidal microorganisms will be an important factor. Engineered microorganisms would self-destruct by expressing a suicide gene after their task is accomplished. These would be developed in response to fears of runaways—that is, harmful genetically engineered microorganisms that rapidly spread destructive power. They would be particularly useful in the bioremediation of solid and hazardous waste sites and in agricultural applications such as fertilizers.

Genetics in Industry

Genetics will first become a force in improving human health, food, and agriculture. But over the next few decades it will have a greater impact across many industries, such as chemical engineering, environmental engineering, manufacturing, energy, and information technology. It will even contribute to the burgeoning field of artificial life.

Chemical engineering, for example, has begun "biologizing"—i.e., incorporating an understanding of complex biological interactions. Genetics will help the chemical industry shift away from bulk chemicals to higher value-added products, such as food additives or industrial enzymes used as biocatalysts.

Genetic engineering will also help to clean the environment and may be used to create totally artificial environments, such as in space and seabed stations or even for terraforming Mars.

Manufacturing, too, will become "biologized" and more like breeding. Manufacturing applications of genetics will include molecular engineering for pharmaceuticals and other compounds, rudimentary DNA chips, biosensors, and nanotechnology based on biological principles such as self-assembly.

A key consideration in biologizing will be society's commitment to sustainability, which could drive a search for environmentally benign manufacturing strategies. Biological approaches, while slower than mechanistic ones, could prove more sustainable. In the future, all industrial enzymes may be produced by genetic engineering. Already, recombinant DNA is used in cheese making, wine making, textiles, and paper production. Bioreactors, in which engineered living cells are used as biocatalysts, will be used for new kinds of manufacturing, such as making new tree species.

Godlike Choices

Even a decision to "let nature run its course" is yet another Godlike choice—albeit one that renounces domains of understanding and control. Such a choice would make us a god of the deists, a passive onlooker of unfolding creation, rather than an active participant in shaping our destiny.

The question, therefore, is not whether we should play God, but what sorts of local gods we will or should become. Will materialism (not the straw man of strong reductionism) demoralize us, or will we continue to find meaning in our personal and social lives even though life itself is understood to be a mechanism? The latter outcome becomes possible if we grasp that our lives' meaning need not depend on our being ethereal, as opposed to purely physical, creatures. Either way, our response to the success of science will help determine how we play the leading role in which nature has cast us on this planet.

Thomas W. Clark, *Humanist*, May 2000.

Linkages may be found between genetics and information technology: Researchers are striving for ways to take advantage of the fact that genes are pure information. A whole new discipline is evolving: "bioinformatics" to manage and interpret the flood of new biological and genomic data. A science of biological computing is also likely to evolve and compete successfully with silicon-based computing.

Genetics and information technology would work together in advanced computers. Biophotonic computers using biomolecules and photonic processors could be the fastest switching systems ever built.

Genetics and Global Development

Genetics could be a tool for igniting a second Green Revolution in agriculture. Synthetic soil supplements, crop strains that accommodate a land's existing conditions, and integrated pest management techniques could be a boon to developing countries, such as India, facing burgeoning population growth on increasingly tired and overworked cropland.

Another potential economic benefit of genetics may be in tourism. Kenya, for instance, could promote tourism associated with wildlife by strengthening its indigenous species. Genetics could be used to rescue lions and elephants from extinction by boosting their food supply or developing vaccines to prevent viral attacks.

Like Kenya, Brazil has an economic opportunity in protecting and enhancing its biodiversity. Brazil's niche would be in pharmaceuticals and other chemicals, and it could tap its lush tropical forests—storehouses of over half the world's plant and animal species. Genes that promote rapid growth could be engineered into the native rain-forest tree species, thus helping to save forests once thought to be lost forever.

Genetics to Improve Human Health

Genetics will increasingly enable health professionals to identify, treat, and prevent the 4,000 or more genetic diseases and disorders that our species is heir to. Genetics will become central to diagnosis and treatment, especially in testing for predispositions and in therapies. By 2025, there will likely be thousands of diagnostic procedures and treatments for genetic conditions.

Genetic diagnostics can detect specific diseases, such as Down's syndrome, and behavioral predispositions, such as depression. Treatments include gene-based pharmaceuticals, such as those using anti-sense DNA to block the body's process of transmitting genetic instructions for a disease process. In future preventive therapies, harmful genes will be removed, turned off, or blocked. In some cases, healthy replacement genes will be directly inserted into fetuses or will be administered to people via injection, inhalation, retroviruses, or pills. These therapies will alter traits and prevent diseases.

Although genetics will be the greatest driver of advances in human health in the twenty-first century, it will not be a panacea for all human health problems. Health is a complex of interacting systems. The benefits of genetics will also be weighted more heavily to future generations, because prevention will be such an important component. Genetic therapies will ameliorate conditions in middle-aged and older people, but those conditions will not even exist in future generations. For example, psoriasis may be brought under control for many via gene therapy; if an effective prenatal diagnosis can be developed, then no future child would ever need be born with the condition.

Genetics and Human Destiny

The greatest genetic challenge of the twenty-first century will be human enhancement. The human species is the first to influence its own evolution. Already, we have seen the use of human growth hormone for more than its original intent as a treatment for dwarfism. In many instances, use of HGH has been cosmetic rather than medically indicated.

In the future, genetics may also be used for mental enhancement. Parents lacking math skills, for example, may shop for genes that predispose their bearer to mathematical excellence and have these genes inserted prenatally or postnatally into their children. Other parents may select traits such as artistic ability, musical talent, charm, honesty, or athletic prowess for their children.

Of course, some challenging social questions are bound to arise as genetics leads to increasingly talented and intelligent children growing up in a society in which they are in many ways superior to their parents, teachers, and government authorities. Optimists may anticipate a more informed and enlightened society. Pessimists would worry about older people being warehoused in communities or homes for the genetically impaired.

"For all the advantages claimed for genetic engineering, in the overwhelming number of cases the price seems too high to pay."

Genetic Engineering Will Not Benefit Society

Ron Epstein

Ron Epstein is a research professor at the Institute for World Religions in Berkeley, California, and a lecturer in philosophy and religion at San Francisco State University. In the following viewpoint, Epstein argues that the short-term benefits of genetic engineering are overshadowed by the long-term negative consequences. For instance, he asserts that attempting to redesign the genetic makeup to improve the human race could result in mistakes that cause irreversible harm to future generations of people. In addition, deadly, fast-moving epidemics could be caused by genetic engineering—either unintentionally or intentionally as an act of biological warfare. Epstein concludes that the mistakes committed through genetic engineering are irreversible.

As you read, consider the following questions:
1. In Epstein's view, what past "scientific miracles" resulted in disaster?
2. Who is James D. Watson? What is his view of genetic engineering?
3. According to Epstein, why does the use of human genes in nonhuman organisms raise ethical questions?

From "Ethical Dangers of Genetic Engineering," by Ron Epstein, *Synthesis/Regeneration*, Fall 1999. Copyright © 1999 by *Synthesis/Regeneration*. Reprinted with permission.

What will it be like in a future world where your life started with your parents designing your genes? In addition to screening for unwanted genetic diseases, they select for sex, height, eye-, hair-, and skin-color. Pressured by the current social fads, they may also choose genes whose overall functions are not clearly understood but are rumored to be connected with temperament, intelligence, mindfulness, and perhaps sexual orientation. You may be genetically engineered to be an enhanced clone of one of your parents, or of a celebrity whose genetic heritage your parents have purchased at great price. If your parents are poor, they may be paid to design you with genes tailored for a particular occupation, together with a pre-birth contract for future employment. As in the film "Gattaca," you probably belong to a clearly defined social class according to the degree of your genetic enhancement. Of course there may still be a few weird, unenhanced naturals-by-choice living in the mountains.

From the very first milk you suckle, your food is genetically engineered. The natural world is completely made over, invaded and distorted beyond recognition by genetically engineered trees, plants, animals, insects, bacteria, and viruses, both planned and run amok. Illnesses are very different too. Most of the old ones are gone or mutated into new forms, yet most people are suffering from genetically engineered pathogens, either used in biowarfare, or mistakenly released into the environment, or recombined in toxic form from originally harmless but rapidly mutating engineered organisms. Genetic engineering is so commonplace, you start your own simple experiments with it in elementary school.

Present Causes Lead to Future Effects

That future is a lot more plausible than you might think. How can it come about? Probably from a combination of misplaced, naïve altruism, the short-sighted quest for short-term corporate profit, power-domination, and just plain emotionally fueled vengeance. In the 1950s, the media were full of information about the great new scientific miracle that was going to make it possible to kill to all of the noxious insects in the world, wipe out insect-borne diseases and feed the world's starving masses. That was DDT [a pesticide that was banned in the United States in 1973 for causing human illness and ecological damage]. In the 1990s, the media are full of information about the coming wonders of genetic engineering. Everywhere are claims that genetic engineering will feed the starving, help eliminate disease, and so forth. The question is the price tag. As has been our experience with most technologies, such as DDT and nuclear energy, the promise of benefit in the short-term is overwhelmed by long-term disasters.

Unlike most other technologies, genetic engineering does not leave room for mistakes. Results of flaws in this technology cannot be recalled and fixed, but become the negative heritage to countless future generations.

In 1976 George Wald, Nobel Prize–winning biologist and Harvard professor, wrote:

> Recombinant DNA technology [genetic engineering] faces our society with problems unprecedented not only in the history of science, but of life on the Earth. It places in human hands the capacity to redesign living organisms, the products of some three billion years of evolution. . . . It presents probably the largest ethical problem that science has ever had to face. Our morality up to now has been to go ahead without restriction to learn all that we can about nature. Restructuring nature was not part of the bargain. . . . For going ahead in this direction may be not only unwise but dangerous. Potentially, it could breed new animal and plant diseases, new sources of cancer, novel epidemics.

Ethical Clarity and Scientific Genius

On the other hand co-discoverer of the DNA code and Nobel laureate Dr. James D. Watson has consistently disregarded the risks of genetic engineering. In 1979 he wrote this about possible diseases that might be inadvertently created through genetic engineering: "I would not spend a penny trying to see if they exist." Claiming that "until a tiger devours you, you don't know that the jungle is dangerous," he wants to plunge forward regardless of the consequences. If Watson wants to go off into the jungle and put himself at risk of being eaten by a tiger, that is his business. When genetically engineered organisms are released into the environment, they put us all at risk, not just their creators. These statements by a great scientist clearly show that we cannot necessarily depend on the high priests of science to make our ethical decisions for us. Too much is at stake.

Yet Watson himself saw some of the problems very clearly when he stated:

> This [genetic engineering] is a matter far too important to be left solely in the hands of the scientific and medical communities. The belief that . . . science always moves forward represents a form of laissez-faire nonsense dismally reminiscent of the credo that American business if left to itself will solve everybody's problems. Just as the success of a corporate body in making money need not set the human condition ahead, neither does every scientific advance automatically make our lives more 'meaningful.'

A Serious Distortion

Although not a geneticist, Stephen Hawking, the renowned physicist and cosmologist, has commented often and publicly on the future role of genetic engineering. One possibility he suggests is that once an intelligent life form reaches the stage we're at now, it proceeds to destroy itself. He's an optimist, however, preferring the notion that people will alter DNA, redesigning the race to minimize our aggressive nature and give us a better chance at long-term survival. "Humans will change their genetic makeup to give them more intelligence and better memory," he said.

If that were the case, why would we be about to destroy ourselves in the first place? Is Hawking assuming that genes control IQ and memory, and that they are equivalent to wisdom, or is Hawking claiming there is a wisdom gene? All these assumptions are extremely dubious. The whole notion that we can completely understand what it means to be human with a small part of our intellect, which is in turn a small part of who we are is, in its very nature, extremely suspect. If we attempt to transform ourselves in the image of a small part of ourselves, what we transform ourselves into will certainly be something smaller or at least a serious distortion of our human nature.

Those questions aside, Hawking does make explicit that for the first time in history, natural evolution has come to an end and has been replaced by human meddling with their own genetic makeup. With genetic engineering science has moved from exploring the natural world and its mechanisms to redesigning them.

Here are some specific examples of ethical problems with the use of genetic engineering.

Biowarfare. It is generally acknowledged that secret work is going forward in many countries to develop genetically engineered bacteria and viruses for biological warfare. International terrorists have already begun seriously considering their use. It is almost impossible to regulate because the same equipment and technology that are used commercially can easily and quickly be transferred to military application.

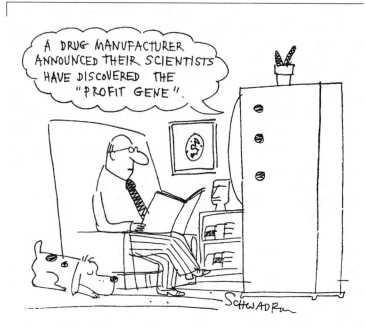

Schwadron. © 2001 by Harley Schwadron. Reprinted with permission.

After reading about the dangers of genetic engineering in biowarfare, the president of the United States, Bill Clinton, became extremely concerned, and, in the spring of 1998, made civil defense countermeasures a priority. Yet his administration has systematically opposed all but the most rudimentary safety regulations and restrictions for the biotech industry. By doing so, Clinton has unwittingly created a climate in which the production of the weapons he is trying to defend against has become very easy for both governments and terrorists.

The former Soviet Union had 32,000 scientists working on biowarfare, including military applications of genetic engineering. No one knows where most of them have gone, or what they have taken with them. Among the more interesting probable developments of their research were smallpox viruses engineered either with equine encephalitis or ebola virus.

Human Genes. As more and more human genes are being inserted into non-human organisms to create new forms of life that are genetically partly human, new ethical questions arise. What percent of human genes does an organism have to contain before it is considered human? For instance, how many human genes would a green pepper have to contain before you would have qualms about eating it? This is not merely a hypothetical query. The Chinese are now putting human genes into tomatoes and peppers to make them grow faster. You can now be a vegetarian and a cannibal at the same time! For meat-eaters, the same question could be posed about eating pork with human genes. What about the mice that have been genetically engineered to produce human sperm? How would you feel if your father was a genetically engineered mouse?

Plastic Plants. So that we would not have to be dependent on petroleum-based plastics, some scientists have genetically engineered plants that produce plastic within their stem structures. They claim that it biodegrades in about six months. If the genes escape into the wild, through cross-pollination with wild relatives or by other means, then we face the prospect of natural areas littered with the plastic spines of decayed leaves. However aesthetically repugnant that may seem, the plastic also poses a real danger. It has the potential for disrupting entire food-chains. It can be eaten by invertebrates, which are in turn eaten, and so forth. If primary foods are inedible or poisonous, then whole food-chains can die off.

Assessing the Price

For all the advantages claimed for genetic engineering, in the overwhelming number of cases the price seems too high to pay. In order to ensure megaprofits for multinational corporations well into the next century, we will have to mortgage the biosphere, seriously compromise life on the planet, and even risk losing what it means to be a human being. Genetic engineering poses serious risks to human health and to the environment. It raises serious ethical questions about the right of human beings to alter life on the planet for the benefit and curiosity of a few.

"The healing potential of genetic testing and treatment could affect literally every symptom we experience."

Genetic Testing Can Benefit Human Health

Emily C. Dossett

In the following viewpoint, Emily C. Dossett contends that genetic testing, the ability to determine if an individual has a genetic predisposition to an illness, can benefit human health. She argues that although there are dangers inherent in genetic testing, such screening can influence people to take control of their own health. Dossett is a medical student in California and a regular contributor to *Sojourners*, a magazine that advocates Christian views on current issues.

As you read, consider the following questions:
1. According to Dossett, which gene is attributed to Huntington's disease?
2. What is Dossett's view of the accessibility of genetic information?
3. According to the author, why is no single person "genetically ideal"?

Everything our bodies need to become whole, healthy, and unique arise from the grand plan contained within one molecule: DNA. The elegance, beauty, and power of God can be seen in the intricacies of human genetics.

Yet not everyone's DNA is perfect—in fact, we all have flaws. Some flaws are not that serious—we may be bow-legged, or gain weight too easily for our liking. But other problems are more profound. Take, for instance, Hunting-ton's Disease. It's caused by a change in the huntingtin gene that one inherits from a parent. Symptoms include a writhing and twisting of the arms, followed by dementia and inevitable death. The disease is not pretty, and there is no treatment.

This is where the dilemmas start. When genetic disorders arise, how far can we go in order to fix them? If we see God in DNA, is it sacred territory? Or are we allowed to ap-proach, to investigate, and to make changes? These are not rhetorical questions. The entire human genome—every bit of DNA—has been mapped out by the Human Genome Project. It's no longer science fiction to use genes to "grow" new organs for transplant, to design medicine that's specific for each individual, or to replace bad genes with new, good ones. Of immediate concern is genetic testing—the ability to determine if a person has genes that will increase or guaran-tee their risk of disease.

Genetic testing holds so much potential for good—and, of course, for bad. A child who has a parent with Hunting-ton's Disease, for example, can be tested to see if he or she has the damaged gene—*but there is no treatment*. All the test yields is the certainty of a horrible, slowly progressing illness that kills at an early age. If there is no treatment, is making such a diagnosis really using the power of genetics to heal?

Not an Unequivocal Evil

Yet genetic testing cannot be written off as an unequivocal evil. For some, there may be comfort in knowledge of what the future holds. And just because we have no treatment for a disease at this time does not mean that we never will. If we were able to use our knowledge of the huntingtin gene to create medicines for those who need it, many lives would be

The Job of Science

It is the job of science, if possible, to develop a vaccine or identify precursors that can take care of disease before it strikes. This is the ideal situation. With genetic screening, many genes associated with diseases have been identified by chromosome location. Therefore, we can determine persons that may have high probabilities of disease or the onset of other characteristics associated with disease. With this we can have preventative medicine, one objective of genetic screening.

Many argue that it is unethical and inhumane to screen persons for disease when there is not a known cure. Treatment of individuals in the past has occurred when the molecular mechanisms of the drugs were not entirely understood. Let screening and treatment of genetic disorders begin while cures are being developed. To withhold this from the public . . . [and] not provide a much-needed service [would be unjust].

Many also argue that it is unethical to implement large screening programs because it infringes on human rights. During the last 20 years, more than 1 million Jews have voluntarily screened for Tay-Sachs. The number of children born with Tay-Sachs has, in many communities, decreased ten-fold. These numbers are obvious to the success of the program.

Another argument against genetic screening is that it could lead to discrimination based on genetics. Discrimination results from public ignorance and fear. This could be facilitated with education and creating programs that are accessible. Just as the confidentiality of our medical records are protected genetic screening test results could also be protected. It only makes sense.

Shannon Oltmans, "Genetic Screening Will Not Put Limits on Equal Opportunity," 1997.

---

saved. Every condition known, from diabetes to heart disease to obesity, has at least some genetic component. Many of these conditions can be altered with diet and exercise, and genetic testing may encourage people to take more control of their health. The healing potential of genetic testing and treatment could affect literally every symptom we experience.

Genetic differences are even more fundamental than the color of our skin, our gender, or where we live, and testing for them could lead to serious discrimination. The results of genetic tests become part of our medical records. Contrary to what we'd like to believe, these records are not really confidential at all, especially with the advent of Web-based medical records; everyone from your insurance agent to your boss can find a way to access them. A person who discovers that he or she has a damaged huntingtin gene could very likely have difficulty finding a job or getting health insurance.

There is a positive side here as well. Every single one of us has genetic mutations—some good, some bad—and there is no single person who is "genetically ideal." One genetic ethicist has predicted that discovery of more and more genetic mutations will naturally lead to national health insurance, since insurance companies will have no one left without a "pre-existing condition" that they are able to cover.

No "Better-than-Thou"

Perhaps the knowledge that there is no "better-than-thou" in genetics will help us realize that we are all equal in the eyes of God and, who knows, maybe some day in each other's eyes as well. God saw infinite possibilities for beauty through one simple molecule, and we are the product of that plan. It is not for us to judge which are more beautiful and to discard the rest, but to appreciate life in all its forms.

"When does [genetic testing] for the benefit of future offspring become confused with eugenics?"

Genetic Testing May Not Benefit Society

Tina Albertson

Genetic testing enables an individual's genetic predisposition to develop a disease or condition to be detected. In the following viewpoint, Tina Albertson contends that although genetic testing is a powerful tool in preventing the onset of numerous illnesses, large-scale testing for genetic disorders may be more harmful than beneficial. For example, Albertson argues that screening the population for diseases may result in high incidences of misdiagnoses. More importantly, she warns that the goal to eliminate harmful genes may lead to eugenics, genetically altering humans for social, racial, or political purposes. Albertson is a biologist and graduate of the University of Oregon at Eugene.

As you read, consider the following questions:
1. Why is genetic control of human diseases highly complex, according to Albertson?
2. According to Albertson, how many genetic mutations that result in cystic fibrosis have been discovered?
3. In the author's view, what nonfatal conditions that can be predicted through genetic testing may lead parents to abort a fetus?

Population screening for genetic disorders, with the intent to eliminate "disease genes" from our population, will be a formidable if not impossible task. The uncertainty in the present screening process will inevitably produce a high incidence of misdiagnoses—through either the failure to detect unique mutations or the detection of false positives—and such mistakes could be devastating to individual lives. Along with these technical arguments, possibly more important to the general public are the ethical arguments against the large-scale genetic screening of the public. If genes for obesity, personality disorders, blindness, or other genes that could be titled "disease genes" are found, should genetic screening with the intent to eliminate this genetic material be legal? And when does screening for the benefit of future offspring become confused with eugenics?

Unavoidable Caveats

There are far too many, as yet unavoidable, caveats in genetic screening to do mass population screening efficiently. As scientists are finding out every day, the genetic control of human disease is much more complicated than anyone could have hoped for. It is being found that very few diseases result from single gene mutations. Most of the prominent fatal genetic disorders such as cancer and heart disease are multigenic, meaning that single mutations in many genes, in varying combinations, can cause one of these complex disorders to manifest. The severity of symptoms also depends on multiple genes, and on how these gene products interact and respond to each other and to the environment. This makes simple genetic tests insufficient to accurately diagnose whether symptoms will arise. Even in disorders that result from a single mutation in a single gene the severity of symptoms cannot be foretold by simply assessing whether the mutation exists. It has been found that some individuals who carry the most common mutation associated with extreme symptoms of cystic fibrosis only exhibit symptoms similar to asthma. This shows that genetic analysis is not adequate as a diagnostic procedure for the severity of disorders that are already genetically defined.

Genetic Discrimination

Genetic discrimination, in the broadest sense, occurs when genetic information is used to treat people differently. In the insurance context, this information may be used to charge higher premiums or refuse people insurance coverage altogether. In the employment setting, genetic information may be used to make decisions about who gets hired, fired, or promoted based on the belief that a genetic marker indicates that an employee will become too sick to work or too costly to insure.

National Partnership for Women and Families, "Genetic Non-Discrimination: Implications for Employers and Employees," July 24, 2001.

It needs to be understood, as scientists are quickly learning, that genes and their products are still enigmas. Each gene is made up of thousands of base pairs that all have the potential to be mutated, and mutations can arise spontaneously all over the genome. Most of the time these mutations are silent: they do not result in dysfunctional gene products. Only when these mutations occur in certain DNA sequences that are essential for normal function of the gene product do genetic diseases occur. It is virtually impossible to design a test that will screen for all permutations that could cause a particular disease because the possible mutations are just too numerous and many are as yet unknown. Taking cystic fibrosis as an example again, 70% of afflicted patients have a particular mutation that would be correctly diagnosed using a current genetic test, another 20% would be correctly diagnosed using a second test, but the remaining 10% would be missed entirely because their mutations are rare or unique. Even those diagnosed with the present tests might be told they carry a debilitating mutation when they may never get sick in their lifetime. With each new test that detects a new mutation there will be a higher risk of misdiagnoses, and since there are now at least 360 known mutations that result in cystic fibrosis, population screening would be a costly and time-consuming process that would not achieve the intended results.

Of course, I am not arguing that genetic screening is not a valuable technique in certain instances. It has certainly been used successfully in diagnosing individual families that are at high risk for Tay-Sachs disease and cystic fibrosis. In these cases fetal screening and pre-implantation screening of embryos are used to avoid the medical and emotional hardships that accompany both of these deadly disorders that onset early in life. But who is going to determine which genetic disorders constitute enough pain and suffering to be eliminated from the population? What about diseases that appear late in life but still allow 40–60 years of productive years of life, as is the case with some cancers and Huntington's disease? Should a fetus be aborted because 60 years later it might die of cancer and in the meantime propagate that same genetic material? Another concern deals with afflictions such as blindness, deafness, or albinism that by some people may be considered diseases. These disorders are not fatal, and rarely even cause pain to the afflicted, but some parents may believe that their child should be spared the emotional hardships that may accompany such genetic conditions. As a result, they may abort a fetus or not allow implantation of these embryos. Is this ethical? I believe these issues must be resolved now, before it turns into a problem of eugenics. Eugenics, with the help of genetic screening, could become a very real and perverse problem in a few years. The line must be drawn between what is legal and right, and what is selfish and wrong. Deadly diseases can be avoided in some cases using this amazing new technology, but this new technology has the potential to be misused. Genetic screening must be used sparingly and at all costs avoid becoming a commercial service that can be exploited.

> "Even if genomic patenting just feels
> morally wrong to some people, it's still
> legally sound."

Scientists Should Be Allowed to Patent Human Genes

Megan Lisagor

In the following viewpoint, Megan Lisagor contends that the patent system is suited to generate the financial resources needed to advance genetic research. If a gene is patented, Lisagor contends, it does not mean that it is owned by one patent holder. Instead, it means that the patent holder has the right to the gene's particular use. Other researchers may use patented gene discoveries if they pay royalties or licensing fees to the patent holder. Lisagor concludes that the public perception of gene patenting is inaccurate and has raised opposition to much-needed patents. Lisagor is a staff writer for the *National Journal*, a weekly magazine on politics, policy, and government.

As you read, consider the following questions:
1. According to Lisagor, how many gene patents were approved by June 2000?
2. How does Lisagor define a "utility" patent, the category under which human DNA is patented?
3. In the author's view, why are gene patents essential to protect the investments of genetic researchers?

The landmark announcement by private and government scientists on June 26, 2000, that they have mapped the entire human genetic code conjures up fearful images of rapacious companies gobbling up patents on this gene or that and selling DNA secrets to the highest bidder. Perhaps an Acme Genetics Co. could corner the market on the gene for blue eyes, or the Blowhard Biotech Co. could nab a patent on blond hair or thinness. In truth, those fears appear to be mostly unfounded, and many scientists and companies in the private and government sectors see the patenting of genes as the best way to prevent a free-for-all when researchers seek rights for using individual genes for new drugs and medical treatments.

Indeed, the U.S. Patent and Trademark Office started patenting genes many years before June 2000's completion of the human genetic blueprint. The agency has already approved more than 1,000 patents for human genes (out of an estimated 50,000 potential patents) and the policy to regulate gene patents is largely settled. That doesn't mean there aren't critics, but even hearings in Congress in July 2000 on new and tougher gene patenting rules are expected to be largely free of controversy since most of industry and academia support the new regulations.

Although gene patenting policy may be clear to scientists, companies, and many lawmakers, it isn't so clear to the public—and sometimes to the media. And that's why even just talking about the issue can cause panic—as it did in the stock market in April 2000 when investors and the media misinterpreted President Clinton and British Prime Minister Tony Blair's comments suggesting that the human genome should be public property. "On the patent thing, you know, Tony Blair and I crashed the market there for a day, and I didn't mean to," Clinton said on April 5, 2000, following the joint statement he made with Blair on gene-based patents. Clinton and Blair were actually endorsing, not questioning, the trademark office's gene patenting policy. The media, however, misunderstood their position, and shareholders lost millions of dollars when their stocks plummeted.

One problem, according to officials and scientists, is that the public's perception of a patent is often wrong. A patent doesn't mean that its holder owns DNA lock, stock, and barrel—it just means that a patent, or a protective right, is issued for a single gene's particular use—its "utility" in patentspeak—not for the discovery of the gene itself. And there's nothing secret about a patent. All U.S. patents are posted on the Patent and Trademark Office's Web site, and other researchers are free to see what utility rights a patentholder has secured on that particular gene. Patent law doesn't preclude others from accessing the isolated gene or its function. It just means that they will probably have to pay royalties or licensing fees to the patentholders who made the discovery. These royalties have become standard practice at biotechnology companies such as Incyte Genomics, the No. 1 carrier of gene patents, which held 316 patents at the end of fiscal 1999. Universities and the federal government, which are committed to sharing information, hold many gene patents, too. The University of California system holds the second most patents, followed by the U.S. Department of Health and Human Services.

The Patent and Trademark Office says that the very old patent laws work well with the very new gene technology. "The same standards of patents since 1952 have allowed us to adapt to new technologies," said Q. Todd Dickinson, the director of the trademark office and undersecretary of Commerce for intellectual property. The Constitution grants Congress power "to promote the progress of science and useful arts, by securing for limited times to authors and inventors the exclusive right to their respective writings and discoveries." Congress enacted the first patent law in 1790. The patent law in effect today dates from 1952 but is essentially a revision of the 1790 act. Section 101 of the 1952 act provides that "anything under the sun" is patentable.

The trademark office is now finalizing new regulations sought by private and federal researchers that will make it harder to get a gene patent. The category of patents that applies to human DNA is "utility" patents. Under the new regulations, according to the patent office, applicants must not only isolate and identify a gene, they must describe its function and how it may be useful for a medical diagnosis or treatment. The guidelines were published in the Federal Register on Dec. 21, 1999, and went through a public comment period that ended on March 22, 2000. The new guidelines were scheduled to be discussed on July 13, 2000, at a hearing before the House Judiciary's Courts and Intellectual Property Subcommittee, and should be finalized by fall 2000.

The Patent System

The leaders in mapping the human genome, J. Craig Venter, the president of Celera Genomics in Rockville, Md., and Francis S. Collins, the director of the National Human Genome Research Institute, which is a part of the National Institutes of Health, praised the patent office's move toward tougher rules. "I think in instances where you have a gene discovery, which has a clear pathway toward a function and a utility that will benefit the public, then the patent system is a good fit for that," Collins said at the June 26, 2000, news conference announcing the completion of the gene mapping project. Venter agreed that the new rules are good. "To get a patent on a gene, you really need to know what the role is going to be: Where is it going to play a role in diagnostics or therapeutics? [It's] not just doing them on economic speculation."

During the public comment period, the majority of organizations submitting statements backed the gene patenting regulations and commended the trademark office for taking steps to "raise the bar" of difficulty in getting gene patents. Some institutions and concerned citizens, however, disagreed strongly—they maintained that no individual or corporation should own human genes. "I want to argue that it's just wrong," said Ben Mitchell, a professor of bioethics and contemporary culture at Trinity University in San Antonio. "Our genes are our common heritage." Mitchell added that the government should explore alternative options to gene patenting that could still protect a company's investments.

And many said that the public has had too few opportunities to air their grievances and worries about gene patenting. Abbey S. Meyers, the president of the National Organization for Rare Disorders, wrote: "Because this topic is so controversial, we have been waiting for the government to initiate a true public dialogue. However, the only opportunities for public input have been responses to the Federal Register notices about proposed rules that are not understandable to ordinary people."

Patent Protection

Nowhere are patents more central to the creative process than in genetic drug development, where human genes and their expressed proteins themselves are developed as therapies. The biotechnology industry in the United States has brought a handful of these crucial new products (recombinant human insulin, to name one of the most familiar) to market and is on the threshold of a bonanza of genetic drugs and vastly greater relief for ill and aging populations around the world.

Patent protection is the sine qua non [absolute prerequisite] of that bonanza. Discovering and developing a new gene-based pharmaceutical product in the United States requires years of commitment and immense capital resources—as much as $500 million. Without the possibility of recouping investment that is bestowed by patents, no biotechnology company would be able to raise the financing necessary to develop these products.

William A. Haseltine, *Technology Review*, September 2000.

Others in the field argue that submitting gene research to patenting and the demands of the marketplace could lead to abuses. Along with Mitchell, opponents of gene patenting say that someone can't own a gene because it's naturally occurring. But John Doll, the director of biotechnology at the trademark office, and private researchers rebut that claim. "It's never existed in that form before," Doll said, referring to the isolated version of the gene, which only happened because a researcher identified it. Chuck Ludlam, vice president for government relations at the Biotechnology Industry Organization, which represents biotechnology companies, academic institutions, and state biotechnology centers, concurs: "You don't own the gene. You have a patent on an industrial invention."

Legally Sound

Even if genomic patenting just feels morally wrong to some people, it's still legally sound, and the new guidelines for gene patenting are so far passing the muster of lawmakers and lawyers. "Our patent laws are the envy of the world and are technologically neutral," said Rep. Howard Coble, R-N.C., who chairs the Courts and Intellectual Property Subcommittee. Coble said he doesn't see a need for new gene patenting legislation.

Bioethicists, however, have less faith in the new patenting guidelines. "I think the rules could be greatly abused," said Gene Rudd, associate director of the Christian Medical & Dental Society. "There are ethical problems. There's no reason to get a patent except for monetary purposes. Profit is the motive."

Rudd is right about the profit motive, which is precisely why the trademark office says that gene patents are necessary. Isolating and identifying genes is a complex and expensive undertaking that takes biotechnology and pharmaceutical companies years to perform. "There's an extraordinary amount of investment that has to be made up front," Dickinson said. Researchers need to earn profits from their investments by finding ways to use genes—usually through drug development. And the drug development process takes additional years of time and money, said Gillian Woollen, associate vice president for biologics and biotechnology at the Pharmaceutical Research and Manufacturers of America (PRMA), which represents approximately 100 U.S. drug companies. Patents grant their owners 20 years of exclusivity that bars others from using their discoveries and allows them to recover their research costs. This exclusivity is essential because the average developmental cost of a drug is now $500 million, according to PRMA.

Venter and Collins, the genome mappers, agree on the role patents play in producing the new medicines that help patients. "One should think of patenting as a method that was put in place to try to make sure that discoveries benefit the public," Collins said. "That's the point. That means that if you've made a discovery that's going to require a substantial investment to bring that product to market, it's a good thing to have a patent around that so that somebody will take a very substantial amount of investment—hundreds of millions of dollars if you are talking about a new drug—and bring that to market without fearing they'll lose their competitive situation the next day."

A Very Key Part

"I think it's very critical to understand that new therapeutics save millions of lives a year," Venter said. "Something as simple and basic as insulin only is available to patients because Genentech and Eli Lilly [and Co.] got a patent for the human insulin gene. So patents are a very key part in the process of making sure new diagnostics and therapeutics get made available to the American public."

Now that the first working drafts of the human genome are assembled, patent applications are pouring in and gene patenting is garnering more attention. "People are justifiably concerned about all this information," said Ludlam, of BIO, but he suggested that once the trademark office's guidelines are official, the controversy will ebb. Still, he acknowledged that "genes are special. There's an emotional edge that makes people react differently." And Coble said the controversy will probably continue as companies compete to make use of the identified genes. "This is the next hot button," Coble said.

"If we patent a human being, we are disregarding that person's intrinsic value."

Scientists Should Not Be Allowed to Patent Human Genes

Julie Narimatsu and Michael Dorsey

Opponents to patenting human genes assert that the inherent value of human life is greater than the need for patents to advance genetic research. In the following viewpoint, Julie Narimatsu and Michael Dorsey suggest that patenting human genes violates human rights by allowing scientists to treat humans as property. In addition, the authors state that many patents are unnecessary because they apply to genes that are neither altered nor useful. Narimatsu is assistant director of the Model United Nations Environmental Progress Committee at the University of Michigan. Dorsey is director of the Sierra Club National Board, an environmental conservation organization.

As you read, consider the following questions:
1. In the authors' opinion, why was John Moore unsuccessful in suing doctors who used his cells to develop a valuable medical discovery?
2. In Narimatsu and Dorsey's view, why did geneticist Noe Zamel travel to the remote island of Tristan da Cunha?
3. According to Narimatsu and Dorsey, how many communities in North America are targeted for gene patenting?

Excerpted from "Playing God or the Work of the Devil: Some Implications of Human Patenting," by Julie Narimatsu and Michael Dorsey, *Synthesis/Regeneration*, Spring 1999. Reprinted with permission.

In 1793, America's first Patent Act was implemented, and the United States Patent Office (USPO) was established. Its curator, Thomas Jefferson, believed that the monopolies that would result from this act were necessary evils that would help make sure that "ingenuity should receive a liberal encouragement." He never would have imagined that 200 years later, society would be in a serious debate over the ability to patent human beings.

In 1985, the USPO decided that all plants, seeds and plant tissues could be patented. Furthermore, in 1987, all living organisms, including animals could be patented. The exclusion of human beings by the Patent Commissioner acknowledged that an ethical issue did exist; nevertheless, body parts, fetuses and embryos are all capable of being patented.

The National Institutes of Health (NIH) has sought patents for DNA fragments from the human genome. Dr. Craig Venter, the man responsible for the sequencing of these fragments, admits that he "still has no idea what it does." The fact that these fragments are currently useless demonstrates the hastiness of NIH and the ignorance of the Patent Office. NIH is not willing to take the time to discover a use unless they are ensured an economic incentive for it. As Dr. Ian Malcolm said, in "Jurassic Park," "You stood on the shoulders of geniuses to accomplish something as fast as you could, and before you even knew what you had, you patented it, packaged it and now you're selling it." The NIH did not discover DNA or the genome, yet they can take credit for "inventing" a part of it.

A Right to Their Own Body Parts?

In 1976, a Seattle businessman named John Moore was treated for a rare form of leukemia at UCLA. The doctors there removed rare "hairy cell leukemia" cells from his spleen. Although Moore signed a standard consent form allowing research on his organ, he was not informed of the commercial value of it. From these cells, the doctors developed antibacterial and cancer-fighting proteins and went on to patent them. They are valued at more than $3 billion. In 1984, Moore sued, claiming that everyone has a right to their own body parts, and that he should be awarded a share of the profits. However, in 1990, the California Supreme Court denied that people have such rights to their bodies. [Philosophy professor] Ned Hettinger explores the rationale that people are "naturally entitled to the fruits of their labor." The Lockean rationale, similarly: "I made it and hence it is mine; it would not have existed but for me." These are the grounds for granting a patent, and, under these rationales, the doctors should not have been granted one. They did not make or create these cells. Had it not been for John Moore, these doctors would not have been able to develop anything at all.

In 1993, the Rural Advancement Foundation International (RAFI) found that the United States had sought U.S. and European patents on a virus from the cells of a 26-year-old Guaymi Indian woman from Panama without her knowledge. Interest in this community strengthened when the NIH discovered that members had a unique virus that may be helpful in AIDS and cancer research. Upon discovery of the activities of the NIH, the Guaymi General Congress protested. The United States ended up withdrawing the NIH's application. However, this incident would not prevent them from trying again.

A Patent-Free Zone

Soon after, the United States applied for two more patents in the U.S. and in Europe. They were interested in cells from peoples of the Solomon Islands and Papua New Guinea. Once again, citizens of these communities protested. The reply came from then Secretary of Commerce, Ron Brown. He stated, "Under our laws, as well as those of many other countries, subject matter relating to human cells is patentable and there is no provision for considerations relating to the sources of the cells that may be the subject of a patent application." In this statement, Brown implied that who and where the human material comes from is irrelevant, and that their protests were futile. This event helped unite several South Pacific Island nations. In March, 1995, the Department of Health and Human Services was granted a patent by the United States Patent Office for the Papua New Guinea Human T-lymphotrophic virus. This was the first human cell line from an indigenous population to be patented. A proposal from the group of nations that included Papua New Guinea established their sovereign space as a "patent-free zone." Subsequently, the United States, once again, abandoned their patent in 1996.

The journey to Tristan da Cunha, often called the world's loneliest island, demonstrates how far these "explorers" would go to find a potential discovery or invention. In April of 1997, Dr. Noe Zamel, a University of Toronto medical geneticist, journeyed by a South African navy ship to this remote island in the middle of the Atlantic Ocean. He was supported by Sequana Therapeutics of La Jolla, California, in the hope of finding genes responsible for asthma. Around half of the island's 300 residents suffer from asthma. From 270 blood samples, his team located two "candidate genes." Until these findings are patented, though, the company is refusing to release any information to any other researchers in this field. They are, thus, accused of putting money in front of finding a cure that would benefit society. This is one example of how much companies are dependent on the patent system to protect their financial interests.

Neither Useful nor Novel

Recently, a U.S. company named Biocyte was awarded a patent by the European Patent Office. This patent applied to all human blood cells from the umbilical cord of a newborn that are used for therapeutic purposes. These cells are a vital part of marrow transplants. Because this patent is so broad, though, Biocyte has the ability to refuse all blood cells from the umbilical cord to anyone who won't pay the fee. Even more ludicrous is the fact that the only reason Biocyte received the patent was because they were able to isolate the cells and deep-freeze them. They did nothing to change or alter them.

Similarly, a company named Systemix was given a patent by the United States Patent Office on all human bone-marrow cells. Again, nothing was altered or changed. We are starting to see a trend where not only does the "invention" not have to be useful, but it doesn't have to be novel, either.

A massive, five year, $35 million project called the Human

Genome Diversity Project seeks to discover all genetic diversity in order to find genes that may be helpful in the development of new drugs. It is run by Dr. Luigi Luca Cavalli-Sforza, a population geneticist and professor at Stanford University and financed by the National Institutes of Health. In order to find these genes, the team will take blood samples, human tissues and hair root from over 10,000 people from 722 indigenous communities. At a cost of $2300 per sample, this $35 million project is more than the per capita GNP [gross national product] of any of the poorest 110 countries. The continuing threat of extinction of these indigenous communities increases the urgency of documenting the genetic makeup of these peoples before they too become extinct. Since 1900, 90 out of the 270 Brazilian indigenous communities have become extinct and more than two-thirds of the remaining communities have less than 1000 members.

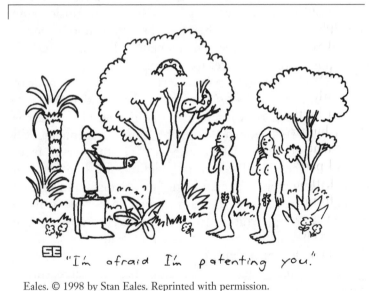

"I'm afraid I'm patenting you."

Eales. © 1998 by Stan Eales. Reprinted with permission.

The targets of this project are spread out somewhat evenly around the world. There are 165 targeted communities in Africa; 212 in Asia; 114 in South America; 101 in Oceania; 107 in North America; and 23 in Europe. In a letter to the National Science Foundation, Tadodaho, chief Leon Shenandoah of the Council of Chiefs of the Onandaga Nation protested, "Your process is unethical, invasive and may even be criminal. It violates the group rights and human rights of our peoples and indigenous peoples around the world. Your project involves the very genetic structures of our beings." In one example, the community of people from Limone in Italy possesses a gene that codes against cardio-vascular disease. This has led to the ambush of this community by Swedish and Swiss pharmaceutical companies and the University of Milan taking blood samples and applying for patents. Have we taken this too far or are the benefits that could potentially come from these patents worth it?

A Person's Intrinsic Value

When we examine the justification of human patenting, we are determining whether or not we value human beings intrinsically. Going back to the nineteenth century, abolitionists argued that every human being had an intrinsic value and "God-given rights." Therefore, humans cannot be made the property of another human being. This argument is valid, but more and more, we are justifying human patents by saying that patents are necessary for the development of anything, even medical treatments and cures derived from human material. We cannot deny that if a cure for cancer is found in the genetic makeup of a human, medicine will greatly benefit from this knowledge. Will the person from whom the genes are taken from benefit at all? The problem is that if we patent a human being, we are disregarding that person's intrinsic value. However, if we do not, we may be giving up an opportunity to save lives. What do we value more? Religious leaders have taken a unanimous stand on the immorality of patenting human life. In May of 1995, a coalition of more than 200 religious leaders, representing every Protestant denomination, Catholicism, Judaism, Islam, Buddhism, and Hinduism, united in the opposition to patenting human genes, organs, tissues and organisms. They did not express opposition to "process" patents to create transgenic life forms, but they concluded that, "Either life is God's creation or a human invention, but it can't be both."

The fact that hundreds of religious leaders from almost all faiths took the same side in this debate says a lot about how religion interprets this issue.

A Frightening Reality

The ownership of a human being by another human being seems preposterous even to modern society yet human patenting has become a frightening reality. From the companies that seek patents to the individuals being sought, the potential for medical breakthroughs is great. How we go about developing these breakthroughs and how we reward them depends on how we value human life. The protests of John Moore and the peoples of New Guinea, Tristan da Cunha and many other indigenous communities around the world have successfully exposed the controversy. Is society prepared to view human life as a mere commercial value? On the other end of the spectrum, the patenting of human life encourages invention and the potential of a medical breakthrough is directly related to this patent system.

From "Jurassic Park," Dr. Ian Malcolm responds to an explanation by one of the scientists about controlling the sex of the dinosaurs to ensure that the dinosaurs did not breed. He says, "If there's one thing the history of evolution has taught us, it's that life will not be contained." We continue to view nature as something we have control over and can manipulate. However, we are now allowing ourselves to be controlled and manipulated. Will the history of evolution prove right? Only the future will tell.

"The Human Genome Project and other genomics research are already having a major impact on research across the life sciences."

Human Genome Research Will Benefit Society

U.S. Department of Energy

In February 2001, scientists announced that they had completed the Human Genome Project, which mapped the entire human genetic code (genome). In the following viewpoint, the U.S. Department of Energy (DOE) claims that human genome research will provide unprecedented insight into human health and illness. The DOE asserts that deciphering the genomic codes of diseases will transform treatments for cancer, Alzheimer's disease, and other serious illnesses. Genome research will greatly enhance the ability to assess the health damage and risks caused by exposure to radiation and carcinogenic toxins. The DOE is a branch of the federal government responsible for overseeing the nation's energy system. It supported the Human Genome Project and is involved in genome research.

As you read, consider the following questions:
1. According to the DOE, what are the major potential applications of genome research?
2. In the author's view, how will molecular medicine be impacted by genome research?
3. In the author's opinion, what are the potential benefits of understanding plant and animal genomes?

Excerpted from "Potential Benefits of Human Genome Project Research," by the U.S. Department of Energy, 2001.

Rapid progress in genome science and a glimpse into its potential applications have spurred observers to predict that biology will be the foremost science of the 21st century. Technology and resources generated by the Human Genome Project and other genomics research are already having a major impact on research across the life sciences. The potential for commercial development of genomics research presents U.S. industry with a wealth of opportunities, and sales of DNA-based products and technologies in the biotechnology industry are projected to exceed $45 billion by 2009.

Some current and potential applications of genome research include

- molecular medicine
- microbial genomics
- risk assessment
- bioarchaeology, anthropology, evolution, and human migration
- DNA forensics (identification)
- agriculture, livestock breeding, and bioprocessing

Molecular Medicine

- *improved diagnosis of disease*
- *earlier detection of genetic predispositions to disease*
- *rational drug design*
- *gene therapy and control systems for drugs*
- *pharmacogenomics "custom drugs"*

Technology and resources promoted by the Human Genome Project are starting to have profound impacts on biomedical research and promise to revolutionize the wider spectrum of biological research and clinical medicine. Increasingly detailed genome maps have aided researchers seeking genes associated with dozens of genetic conditions, including myotonic dystrophy, fragile X syndrome, neurofibromatosis types 1 and 2, inherited colon cancer, Alzheimer's disease, and familial breast cancer.

On the horizon is a new era of molecular medicine characterized less by treating symptoms and more by looking to the most fundamental causes of disease. Rapid and more specific diagnostic tests will make possible earlier treatment of countless maladies. Medical researchers also will be able to devise novel therapeutic regimens based on new classes of drugs, immunotherapy techniques, avoidance of environmental conditions that may trigger disease, and possible augmentation or even replacement of defective genes through gene therapy.

Microbial Genomics

- *new energy sources (biofuels)*
- *environmental monitoring to detect pollutants*
- *protection from biological and chemical warfare*
- *safe, efficient toxic waste cleanup*
- *understanding disease vulnerabilities and revealing drug targets*

In 1994, taking advantage of new capabilities developed by the genome project, the U.S. Department of Energy (DOE) initiated the Microbial Genome Program to sequence the genomes of bacteria useful in energy production, environmental remediation, toxic waste reduction, and industrial processing.

Despite our reliance on the inhabitants of the microbial world, we know little of their number or their nature: estimates are that less than 0.01% of all microbes have been cultivated and characterized. Programs like the DOE Microbial Genome Program (MGP) help lay a foundation for knowledge that will ultimately benefit human health and the environment. The economy will benefit from further industrial applications of microbial capabilities.

Information gleaned from the characterization of complete genomes in MGP will lead to insights into the development of such new energy-related biotechnologies as photosynthetic systems, microbial systems that function in extreme environments, and organisms that can metabolize readily available renewable resources and waste material with equal facility. Expected benefits also include development of diverse new products, processes, and test methods that will open the door to a cleaner environment. Biomanufacturing will use nontoxic chemicals and enzymes to reduce the cost and improve the efficiency of industrial processes. Already, microbial enzymes are being used to bleach paper pulp, stone wash denim, remove lipstick from glassware, break down starch in brewing, and coagulate milk protein for cheese production. In the health arena, microbial sequences may help researchers find new human genes and shed light on the disease-producing properties of pathogens.

Opening Up the Genome

The Human Genome Initiative began in the late 1980s, an outgrowth of discussions among scientists from multiple disciplines—initially met with considerable skepticism—about the possibility of deciphering the entire genetic makeup of Homo sapiens. In the spring of 1987, the Health and Environmental Research Advisory Committee of the US Department of Energy prepared *The Report of the Human Genome Initiative*, and the following year the Office of Technology Assessment published a detailed analysis of the scientific advances that might equip the research community to undertake the project. Congress then appropriated funds to the US Department of Energy and the National Institutes of Health earmarked for research into the study of complex genomes.

With the overall intent of furthering the basic scientific understanding of human genetics and the role of genes in health and disease, the project's initial goals were

- Construction of a high-resolution genetic map of the human genome.
- Production of a variety of physical maps of all human chromosomes and of the DNA of selected model organisms, with emphasis on maps that make the DNA accessible to investigators for further analysis. This series of maps would be of increasingly fine resolution.
- Determination of the complete sequence of human DNA and DNA of selected model organisms.

Nancy Walsh D'Eperio, *Patient Care*, November 15, 1998.

Microbial genomics will also help pharmaceutical researchers gain a better understanding of how pathogenic microbes cause disease. Sequencing these microbes will help reveal vulnerabilities and identify new drug targets.

Gaining a deeper understanding of the microbial world also will provide insights into the strategies and limits of life on this planet. Data generated in this young program already have helped scientists identify the minimum number of genes necessary for life and confirm the existence of a third major kingdom of life. Additionally, the new genetic techniques now allow us to establish more precisely the diversity of microorganisms and identify those critical to maintaining or restoring the function and integrity of large and small ecosystems; this knowledge also can be useful in monitoring and predicting environmental change. Finally, studies on microbial communities provide models for understanding biological interactions and evolutionary history.

Risk Assessment

- *assess health damage and risks caused by radiation exposure, including low-dose exposures*
- *assess health damage and risks caused by exposure to mutagenic chemicals and cancer-causing toxins*
- *reduce the likelihood of heritable mutations*

Understanding the human genome will have an enormous impact on the ability to assess risks posed to individuals by exposure to toxic agents. Scientists know that genetic differences make some people more susceptible and others more resistant to such agents. Far more work must be done to determine the genetic basis of such variability. This knowledge will directly address DOE's long-term mission to understand the effects of low-level exposures to radiation and other energy-related agents, especially in terms of cancer risk.

Human Evolution and Biology

- *study evolution through germline mutations in lineages*
- *study migration of different population groups based on female genetic inheritance*
- *study mutations on the Y chromosome to trace lineage and migration of males*
- *compare breakpoints in the evolution of mutations with ages of populations and historical events*

Understanding genomics will help us understand human evolution and the common biology we share with all of life. Comparative genomics between humans and other organisms such as mice already has led to similar genes associated with diseases and traits. Further comparative studies will help determine the yet-unknown function of thousands of other genes.

Comparing the DNA sequences of entire genomes of different microbes will provide new insights about relationships among the three kingdoms of life: archaebacteria, eukaryotes, and prokaryotes.

DNA Forensics

- *identify potential suspects whose DNA may match evidence left at crime scenes*
- *exonerate persons wrongly accused of crimes*
- *identify crime and catastrophe victims*
- *establish paternity and other family relationships*
- *identify endangered and protected species as an aid to wildlife officials (could be used for prosecuting poachers)*
- *detect bacteria and other organisms that may pollute air, water, soil, and food*
- *match organ donors with recipients in transplant programs*
- *determine pedigree for seed or livestock breeds*
- *authenticate consumables such as caviar and wine*

Any type of organism can be identified by examination of DNA sequences unique to that species. Identifying individuals is less precise at this time, although when DNA sequencing technologies progress further, direct characterization of very large DNA segments, and possibly even whole genomes, will become feasible and practical and will allow precise individual identification.

To identify individuals, forensic scientists scan about 10 DNA regions that vary from person to person and use the data to create a DNA profile of that individual (sometimes called a DNA fingerprint). There is an extremely small chance that another person has the same DNA profile for a particular set of regions.

Agriculture, Livestock Breeding, and Bioprocessing

- *disease-, insect-, and drought-resistant crops*
- *healthier, more productive, disease-resistant farm animals*
- *more nutritious produce*
- *biopesticides*
- *edible vaccines incorporated into food products*
- *new environmental cleanup uses for plants like tobacco*

Understanding plant and animal genomes will allow us to create stronger, more disease-resistant plants and animals—reducing the costs of agriculture and providing consumers with more nutritious, pesticide-free foods. Already growers are using bioengineered seeds to grow insect- and drought-resistant crops that require little or no pesticide. Farmers have been able to increase outputs and reduce waste because their crops and herds are healthier.

Alternate uses for crops such as tobacco have been found. One researcher has genetically engineered tobacco plants in his laboratory to produce a bacterial enzyme that breaks down explosives such as TNT and dinitroglycerin. Waste that would take centuries to break down in the soil can be cleaned up by simply growing these special plants in the polluted area.

"[Human genome research] is a major diversion and obstruction, and is preventing us from addressing the overwhelming environmental and social causes of ill-health."

Human Genome Research Will Not Benefit Society

Mae-Wan Ho

Completed in February 2001, the Human Genome Project was commenced by scientists in 1987 in order to decipher the entire human genetic code (genome). Supporters claim that the project will revolutionize medicine. In the following viewpoint, Mae-Wan Ho argues that human genome research is useless. Ho contends geneticists are baffled by the genome sequences they have discovered and will not produce any medical breakthroughs. She insists that instead of investigating the human genome, medical research must focus on countering the environmental and social causes of human diseases. Ho is founder and director of the Institute of Science in Society (I-SIS), a nonprofit organization based in London, England, that seeks to maintain social responsibility within the fields of scientific research and application.

As you read, consider the following questions:

1. According to Ho, what percent of human diseases can be attributed to genetics alone?
2. What is Ho's opinion of antibiotics?
3. In the author's view, what characterizes a holistic approach to health care?

Excerpted from Mae-Wan Ho's speech "The Human Genome—A Big White Elephant," delivered at the Green Research Forum, European Parliament, Brussels, Austria, June 6, 2001. Copyright © 2001 by www.i-sis.org. Reprinted with permission.

The human genome may go down in history as the biggest white elephant for humanity. It cost a lot and is useless, it does not work, and is so expensive to maintain and grows so big so fast that it will bankrupt the industry as well as entire nations. The only clear message in the 'book of life' is "there is no one home, life is not to be found here." Craig Venter, whose company Celera raced the publicly funded sequencing consortium to the finishing line, said as much, "We simply do not have enough genes for this idea of biological determinism to be right. The wonderful diversity of the human species is not hard-wired in our genetic code. Our environments are critical."

I was a researcher and lecturer in genetics throughout the mid-1970s to the early 1980s when new discoveries on the fluid genome made headlines every week, overturning the most deeply held convictions of classical genetics. Craig Venter may have just discovered that genetic determinism cannot deliver the goods, after sequencing the human genome. But many of us knew that genetic determinism had died with the revelations of the fluid genome, if not before.

The scientific establishment has remained firmly wedded to genetic determinism, if only because it is indispensable for business. It is also fuelling the resurgence of eugenics and genetic discrimination, and making even the most unethical uses seem compelling, such as the creation of human embryos to supply cells and tissues for transplant in so-called 'therapeutic' human cloning.

I started my career in human biochemical genetics, studying genuine genetic diseases that could be attributed to mutations in single genes. These account for no more than 2% of all human ailments. But diagnosing and curing rare single gene defects simply "did not fit the business model." So, 'genetic defects' and 'gene therapy' expanded in recent years to include the far more common and potentially highly profitable diseases such as cancer, heart disease, AIDS, Alzheimer's and Parkinson's. Francis Collins, head of the public human genome consortium, runs a laboratory in the US National Institutes of Health. He is now engaged in a "huge and very complicated" search for genes for adult-onset diabetes. Adult-onset diabetes, like asthma and cancer has reached epidemic proportions over the years, increasing from 4.9% in 1990 to 6.5% in 1998, in both sexes, across all ages, ethnic groups, education levels, and in nearly all states in the United States. That should have alerted all rational scientists to look for environmental causes instead of genes.

The Genetic Determinist Myth

James Watson and other proponents of the human genome project perpetrated the ultimate genetic determinist myth that the human genome sequence contains the 'blueprint for making a human being.' The public has paid out billions of dollars in the United States and hundreds of millions of pounds in the United Kingdom. Now, dozens of genome sequences later, the sequencers haven't a clue of how to make the smallest bacterium or the simplest worm, let alone a human being. The human genome may consist of up to 98.9% 'junk DNA' with no known function. Geneticists are baffled. [According to Tom Bethell], "The genome isn't a code, and we can't read it."

Public investment was needed to keep the human genome in the public domain, we were told. But that had not prevented any human gene from being patented. On the contrary, scientists funded by the public have been busy patenting genes and starting up private companies, with little or no return to the public coffers. Genes and cell lines stolen from indigenous peoples are patented, and governments are selling DNA databases of entire nations to private companies. These patents and proprietary databases not only violate basic human rights and dignity, they are seriously distorting healthcare and stifling scientific research and innovation. They should be firmly rejected by the scientific community.

Now, the elephant attendants are saying the human genome needs more money before it can deliver the goods. The UK Government is obligingly giving away £2.5 billion over the next four years to 'health genomics,' to identify all the genes that predispose the UK population to disease. The elephant is growing big fast.

Such massive divestments of public funds are designed to bail out the biotech industry already in trouble over genetically modified (GM) crops, and now showing every sign of being driven bankrupt by the human genome. But the real disaster will fall on public health. It is narrowing the options for healthcare and foreclosing other promising approaches. Health genomics is a major diversion and obstruction, and is preventing us from addressing the overwhelming environmental and social causes of ill-health. It will also victimise those most in need of care and treatment. I call it 'a scientific and financial black hole,' a colossal waste of scientific imagination and financial resources.

The Failures of Reductionist Medicine

In many respects, health genomics epitomises the failures of reductionist medicine, which have reached crisis proportions. Drug and antibiotic resistant infectious diseases have come back with a vengeance within the past 25 years. Infectious diseases are responsible for one-quarter of the 53.9 million deaths in the world, second to cardiovascular disease. For poor countries and children under five, however, infectious diseases top the list, accounting respectively for 45% and 63% of deaths. Among the factors blamed are the overuse and abuse of antibiotics, destruction of the environment, poverty, malnutrition and increase in air travel, all of which serves to remind us that disease cannot be understood in reductionist terms. One likely contributing factor that has yet to be named by the scientific establishment is the rise of commercial genetic engineering within the same period. Genetic engineering, in agriculture as in medicine, uses the same tools and makes the same kinds of artificial constructs, all of which enhance horizontal gene transfer and recombination, precisely the processes that create new pathogens and spread drug and antibiotic resistance genes.

The other big killers are cardiovascular disease, which tops the list at 31%, and cancer at 13%, after infectious diseases. Both cardiovascular disease and cancer are predominantly illnesses of rich industrialised nations. Cancers are linked to ionising radiation and to the hundreds of actual and potential carcinogens among the industrial and agricultural chemicals polluting our air, water and soil.

The incidence of cancer is known to increase with industrialisation and pesticide use. Women in non-industrial

Asian countries have a much lower incidence of breast cancer compared to women living in the industrialised west. However, when Asian women emigrate to Europe and the United States, their incidence of cancer jumps to that of the white European women within a single generation. Similarly, when DDT and other pesticides were phased out in Israel, breast cancer mortality in pre-menopausal women dropped by 30%. Environmental influences clearly swamp out even large genetic differences.

Health genomics research will do nothing to identify or remove the causes of cancer. Instead, it will identify all the genes that 'predispose' the victims to cancers, to enable corporations that have made lots of money polluting the environment with carcinogens to make lots more money selling diagnostic tests and 'miracle cures.' Patients are bankable assets, and terminal cancer patients all the more so.

The Cures May Be Far Worse

The disease statistics are bad enough. But the cures may be far worse. Successive studies have documented a rising epidemic of iatrogenic diseases, ie, diseases caused by medical treatments, interventions and drugs. Doctors are now the third leading cause of death in the US, responsible for some 250,000 every year, among which are 106,000 due to non-error negative effects of drugs. The problem is not confined to the US; it is endemic in all industrialised countries that adhere to the same reductionist model of health and disease: Canada, Australia, New Zealand and Britain. We can already see the tip of the iceberg in the new classes of iatrogenic diseases that 'health genomics' will bring. Clinical trials of 'gene therapy' have killed six and caused more than 650 adverse events. The 'miracle cure' for Parkinson's turned into an irredeemable nightmare because the cells from foetuses transplanted into five patients' brains grew uncontrollably. And watch out for viral pandemics if xenotransplantation [animal-to-human organ transplants] is to go ahead.

A sweeping paradigm change is long overdue. The human genome, like the genome of any other organism, is fluid and dynamic. Genes function organically, in entangled networks that respond from moment to moment to the changing context of the whole organism in its ecosystem. They are not mechanical elements operating in fixed circuit boards. Let me give a few recent examples of how genes, genomes and organisms respond organically to their environment, demanding a radical rethink of the conventional approach.

Many bacteria are now found to change reversibly from a benign, non-proliferative phase to a pathogenic, proliferative phase, depending on ecological conditions. Some scientists are now rethinking the failed conventional model of killing pathogens with new, ever more deadly antibiotics as bacteria become resistant to the old ones. They are designing drugs that physiologically tame the bacteria, rather than kill them. A logical extension of that approach is to find how ecological balance could be achieved, so bacteria do not become virulent.

Knowing Is Not Understanding

To know the sequence of the human genome is not the same as understanding it or finding the cure for cancer. Men can map the moon in some detail, but they cannot live there. . . . The idea that there are genes "for" particular diseases, and all we have to do is to turn them "off", is naive. Worse still is the belief—because it has such dangerous social implications—that there are genes for homosexuality, criminality, intelligence, heroin addiction and so on. It takes whole groups of interacting genes to produce particular effects; the same genes, under different environmental conditions, will act differently and produce different effects.

New Statesman, July 3, 2000.

The dominant reductionist model of cancer says cancer is caused by mutations in specific cancer genes and cancer-suppressing genes. There is growing evidence that those gene mutations are neither necessary nor sufficient for cancer to develop. Every cancer has a different genetic signature. In fact, every cancerous growth in an individual differs in genetic signature. The cancerous state is a physiological response of the cell to its environment, which is ultimately the whole organism in its ecological context. Cancer is associated with gross genetic instability that gives rise to large genomic abnormalities. Cancer cures based on single molecular interventions offered by health genomics will therefore be largely irrelevant and ineffective. The emphasis must be prevention rather than cure. The phenomenon of spontaneous cancer remission should also be much more thoroughly investigated. Remissions can occur after various experiences that affect the whole body, such as fever, a change of diet or change of life-style.

There have been a large number of observations suggesting that genes in bacteria and other organisms can mutate in response to environmental challenges, so as to enable them to survive. There is evidence that defective genes in human beings can also regain function by mutation. Cells in the body of individuals born with defective genes have been found to revert spontaneously to functional states. Thus, rather than persist in futile and dangerous attempts at 'gene therapy,' substantial effort ought to be redirected towards elucidating the physiological and environmental conditions that can encourage the body to mend its own defective genes.

Aiming at the Organic Whole

We have had decades, if not centuries, of reductionist, mechanistic science that has given us a surfeit of knowledge of the parts, not all of which has been put to good, sustainable use. Now is the time to complement this knowledge of the parts with investigations aimed at knowledge of the organic whole that can truly bring health and well being to the community. In particular, I propose that we target at least part of our research budget to the following areas which are currently either grossly under-funded, or not funded at all.

1. Ecology and Energy Use in Sustainable Systems
- To investigate the precise role of complexity and biodiversity
- To elucidate energy-relationships, energy use, renewable energies
- To identify biophysical indicators of ecosystem health
- To develop non-invasive, non-destructive technologies for monitoring and regulating environmental quality

2. Science of the Organism and Holistic Health
- To articulate a concept of an organic whole as the basis of health

- To identify biophysical and dynamical indicators of health
- To develop non-invasive, non-destructive technologies for monitoring health and for quality control of food and other agricultural produce
- To develop effective therapeutic methods based on minimum intervention

3. Working Science Partnerships
- To enable scientists to work directly with local communities
- To revitalise and protect traditional agricultural and healthcare systems from biopiracy and globalisation
- To develop appropriate sciences and technologies

4. Science and Technology Monitor
- To monitor new developments for social/ecological accountability and safety
- To promote critical public understanding
- To promote science-public dialogue and public participation.

Periodical Bibliography

The following articles have been selected to supplement the diverse views presented in this chapter. Addresses are provided for periodicals not indexed in the *Readers' Guide to Periodical Literature*, the *Alternative Press Index*, the *Social Sciences Index*, or the *Index to Legal Periodicals and Books*.

Garland E. Allen	"Is a New Eugenics Afoot?" *Science*, October 5, 2001.
Stephen A. Bent and Qin Shi	"Patenting Genes: The New Frontier," *National Law Review*, March 6, 2000.
Nell Boyce	"Redesigning Dad," *U.S. News & World Report*, November 5, 2001.
Larry R. Churchill	"We Are Our Genes—Not," *World & I*, November 2001.
Steve Connor	"Q: How Close Are We to Unlocking the Secret Code of Life? A: Close, Very Close," *Independent*, February 12, 2001.
Frederic Golden	"Good Eggs, Bad Eggs: The Growing Power of Prenatal Genetic Tests Is Raising Thorny New Questions About Ethics, Fairness, and Privacy," *Time*, January 11, 1999.
William A. Haseltine	"In Gene Patents, We're the Champ," *Wall Street Journal*, March 9, 2000.
Neil A. Holtzman and Theresa M. Marteau	"Will Genetics Revolutionize Medicine?" *New England Journal of Medicine*, July 13, 2000.
Wil S. Hylton	"Who Owns This Body?" *Esquire*, July 2001.
Los Angeles Times	"Taming Gene Patent Gold Rush," May 22, 2000.
Sheila McLean	"Genetic Screening—Controlling the Future," *Biological Sciences Review*, March 2000.
Andrew Sullivan	"Promotion of the Fittest," *New York Times Magazine*, July 23, 2000.
Nicholas Wade	"Human Genome Appears More Complicated," *New York Times*, August 24, 2001.
Wall Street Journal	"Of Genomes and Governments," February 13, 2001.
Adam Wolfson and Ronald Baily	"Does Genetic Engineering Endanger Human Freedom?" *American Enterprise*, October 2001.

For Further Discussion

Chapter 1

1. Nathan Myhrvold and Wesley J. Smith address the risk of discrimination in their arguments regarding human cloning. How are their arguments about discrimination similar? How are they different? Whose argument is more persuasive, and why?

2. According to John F. Kilner, supporters justify human cloning on the basis of utility: People can be justly used as a means to an end. In your opinion, is the Human Cloning Foundation's argument for human cloning based on utility? Why or why not?

Chapter 2

1. Richard A. Epstein argues that offering organ donors payment for their organs will increase the supply of organs for transplant. On the other hand, James F. Childress maintains that the sale of organs will worsen the organ shortage. Who makes the stronger argument? Explain your answer.

2. Melanie Phillips asserts that presumed consent for organ donation hands over people's bodies to the government. In your opinion, do the presumed consent policies that I. Kennedy and others explore treat people's bodies as the government's property? Why or why not?

Chapter 3

1. In your view, does Dion Farquhar successfully counter Janice G. Raymond's argument that reproductive technologies are wholly unethical because they harm women? Explain your answer.

2. Lawrence A. Kalikow insists that surrogate motherhood allows couples to express their procreative freedom. However, Scott B. Rae maintains that surrogacy is oppressive because it constitutes the sale of children. In your opinion, who makes the stronger argument? Provide examples from the viewpoints to support your answer.

Chapter 4

1. Ron Epstein claims that genetic engineering offers humanity only "short-term" benefits. In your opinion, do Joseph F. Coates, John B. Mahaffie, and Andy Hines offer only short-term benefits of genetic engineering? Provide examples from the viewpoint in your answer.

2. Emily C. Dossett and Tina Albertson both address the possibility of receiving devastating genetic test results. How are their

arguments different? In your view, who makes the more compelling argument?

3. Mae-Wan Ho argues that the Human Genome Project has diverted attention from the environmental causes of diseases. Do you believe that the U.S. Department of Energy acknowledges these causes of disease in their viewpoint supporting the Human Genome Project? Why or why not?

Organizations to Contact

The editors have compiled the following list of organizations concerned with the issues debated in this book. The descriptions are derived from materials provided by the organizations. All have publications or information available for interested readers. The list was compiled on the date of publication of the present volume; the information provided here may change. Be aware that many organizations take several weeks or longer to respond to inquiries, so allow as much time as possible.

American Anti-Vivisection Society
801 Old York Rd., Suite 204, Jenkintown, PA 19046-1685
(215) 887-0816 • fax: (215) 887-2088
e-mail: aavsonline@aol.com • website: www.aavs.org

The oldest animal rights group in America, the American Anti-Vivisection Society opposes all animal experimentation. It publishes educational pamphlets and the quarterly *AV Magazine*.

American Civil Liberties Union (ACLU)
125 Broad St., 18th Floor, New York, NY 10004-2400
(212) 549-2500 • publications: (800) 775-ACLU (2258)
e-mail: aclu@aclu.org • website: www.aclu.org

The ACLU champions civil rights protected by the U.S. Constitution. The union is concerned that genetic testing may lead to genetic discrimination in the workplace, including the refusal to hire and desire to terminate employees who are at risk for developing genetic conditions. The ACLU publishes a variety of handbooks, pamphlets, reports, and newsletters, including the quarterly *Civil Liberties* and the monthly *Civil Liberties Alert*.

American Medical Association (AMA)
515 N. State St., Chicago, IL 60610
(312) 464-5000
website: www.ama-assn.org

The AMA is the largest professional association for medical doctors. It helps set standards for medical education and practices and it is a powerful lobby in Washington, D.C., for physicians' interests. The association publishes journals for many medical fields, including the monthly *Archives of Surgery* and the weekly *JAMA*.

American Society of Law, Medicine, and Ethics (ASLME)
765 Commonwealth Ave., 16th Floor, Boston, MA 02215
(617) 262-4990 • fax: (617) 437-7596
e-mail: aslme@bu.edu • website: www.aslme.org

The ASLME's members include physicians, attorneys, health care administrators, and others interested in the relationships between law, medicine, and ethics. It takes no positions but acts as a forum for discussion of issues such as genetic engineering. The organization has an information clearinghouse and a library. It publishes the quarterlies *American Journal of Law & Medicine* and *Journal of Law, Medicine & Ethics*.

Biotechnology Industry Organization (BIO)
1225 Eye St. NW, Suite 400, Washington, DC 20005
(202) 962-9200
e-mail: info@bio.org • website: www.bio.org

The BIO is composed of companies engaged in industrial biotechnology. It monitors government actions that affect biotechnology and promotes increased public understanding of biotechnology through its educational activities and workshops. The BIO is committed to the socially responsible use of biotechnology to save or improve lives, improve the quality and abundance of food, and clean up hazardous waste. It publishes online bulletins and the bimonthly newsletter *BIO News*.

Childbirth by Choice Trust
344 Bloor St. W., Suite 502, Toronto, ON, M5S 3A7, CANADA
(416) 961-7812
e-mail: cbctrust@idirect.com • website: www.cbctrust.com

The Childbirth by Choice Trust aims to educate the public on fertility control issues, such as contraceptive use, abortion, and unintended pregnancy. It hopes to make all options available to women who are unhappily pregnant, including abortion, childbirth, and adoption. The trust provides educational pamphlets that provide information about fertility control issues, such as *Abortion: The Medical Procedure, Contraceptive Use in Canada*, and *Economics of Unintended Pregnancy*. These pamphlets can be ordered through their website or by mail.

Council for Responsible Genetics
5 Upland Rd., Suite 3, Cambridge, MA 02140
(617) 868-0870 • fax: (617) 491-5344
e-mail: crg@essential.org • website: www.gene-watch.org

The Council for Responsible Genetics is a national organization of scientists, health professionals, trade unionists, women's health activists, and others who work to ensure that biotechnology is developed safely and in the public interest. The council publishes the bimonthly newsletter *GeneWatch* and position papers on the Human Genome Project, genetic discrimination, germ-line modifications, and DNA-based identification systems.

The Hastings Center
Garrison, NY 10524-5555
(914) 424-4040 • fax: (914) 424-4545
e-mail: mail@thehastingscenter.org
website: www.thehastingscenter.org

Since it was founded in 1969, the Hastings Center has played a central role in responding to the ethical questions raised by advances in medicine and biotechnology. It conducts research on such issues and provides consultations. The center publishes books, papers, guidelines, and the bimonthly *Hastings Center Report*.

National Bioethics Advisory Commission (NBAC)
6100 Executive Blvd., Suite 5B01, Rockville, MD 20592-7508
(301) 402-4242 • fax: (301) 480-6900
website: www.bioethics.gov

The NBAC is a federal agency that sets guidelines to govern the ethical conduct of biotechnological research. It works to protect the rights and welfare of human research subjects and oversee the management and use of genetic information. Its published reports include *Cloning Human Beings* and *Ethical Issues in Human Stem Cell Research*.

National Institutes of Health (NIH)
National Human Genome Research Institute (NHGRI)
9000 Rockville Pike, Bethesda, MD 20892
(301) 402-0911 • fax: (301) 402-0837
website: www.nhgri.nih.gov

The NIH is the federal government's primary agency for the support of biomedical research. As a division of the NIH, the NHGRI's mission is to head the Human Genome Project, the federally funded effort to map all human genes. Information about the Human Genome Project is available at the NHGRI's website.

United Network for Organ Sharing (UNOS)
1100 Boulders Pkwy., Suite 500, Richmond, VA 23225
(804) 330-8500 • fax: (804) 330-8507
website: www.unos.org

UNOS is a system of transplant and organ procurement centers, tissue-typing labs, and transplant surgical teams. It was formed to match organ donors with people in need of organs. By law, organs used for transplants must be cleared through UNOS. The network also formulates and implements national policies on equal access to organs and organ allocation, organ procurement, and AIDS testing. It publishes the quarterly *UNOS Update*.

Bibliography of Books

Brian Appleyard — *Brave New Worlds: Staying Human in the Genetic Future*. New York: Viking, 1998.

Arthur L. Caplan and Daniel H. Coelho, eds. — *The Ethics of Organ Transplants: The Current Debate*. Amherst, NY: Prometheus Books, 1998.

Jeremy R. Chapman, Mark Deierhio, and Celia Wight, eds. — *Organ and Tissue Donation for Transplantation*. New York: Edward Arnold, 1997.

Ronald Cole-Turner — *Human Cloning: Religious Perspectives*. Louisville, KY: Westminster John Knox, 1997.

Ann Donchin and Laura M. Purdy, eds. — *Embodying Bioethics: Recent Feminist Advances*. Lanham, MD: Rowman & Littlefield, 1999.

Jeanette Edwards et al. — *Technologies of Procreation: Kinship in the Age of Assisted Reproduction*. New York: Routledge, 1999.

Kay Elder and Brian Dale, eds. — *In Vitro Fertilization*. New York: Cambridge University Press, 2000.

Michael W. Fox — *Beyond Evolution: The Genetically Altered Future of Plants, Animals, the Earth—and Humans*. New York: Lyons Press, 1999.

Sarah Franklin — *Embodied Progress: A Cultural Account of Assisted Reproduction*. New York: Routledge, 1997.

D.J. Galton — *In Our Own Image: Eugenics and the Genetic Modification of People*. London: Little, Brown, 2001.

James M. Humber and Robert F. Almeder, eds. — *Human Cloning*. Totowa, NJ: Humana Press, 1998.

Margaret O. Hyde and John Setaro — *When the Brain Dies First*. New York: Franklin Watts, 2000.

Maureen Junker-Kenny, ed. — *Designing Life?: Genetics, Procreation, and Ethics*. Brookfield, VT: Ashgate, 1999.

Arlene Judith Klotzko, ed. — *The Cloning Sourcebook*. New York: Oxford University Press, 2001.

Paul Lauritzen, ed. — *Cloning and the Future of Human Embryo Research*. New York: Oxford University Press, 2001.

Margaret Lock — *Twice Dead: Organ Transplants and the Reinvention of Death*. Berkeley and Los Angeles: University of California Press, 2001.

Richard Lynn — *Eugenics: A Reassessment*. Westport, CT: Praeger 2001.

Barbara MacKinnon, ed.	*Human Cloning: Science, Ethics, and Public Policy.* Urbana: University of Illinois Press, 2000.
Glenn McGee, ed.	*The Human Cloning Debate.* Berkeley, CA: Berkeley Hills Books, 2000.
Martha C. Nussbaum and Cass R. Sunstein, eds.	*Clones and Clones: Facts and Fantasies About Human Cloning.* New York: Norton, 1998.
Louis J. Palmer	*Organ Transplants from Executed Prisoners: An Argument for the Creation of Death Sentence Removal Statutes.* Jefferson, NC: MacFarland, 1999.
M.L. Rantala and Arthur J. Milgram, eds.	*Cloning: For and Against.* Chicago: Open Court, 1999.
Jeremy Rifkin	*The Biotech Century.* New York: Jeremy P. Tarcher/Putnam, 1998.
R.G. Rosdan	*Designing Babies: The Brave New World of Reproductive Technologies.* New York: W.H. Freeman, 1999.
Ann Rudinow Saetnan, Nelly Oudshoorn, and Marta Kirejczyk, eds.	*Bodies of Technology: Women's Involvement with Reproductive Medicine.* Columbus: Ohio State University Press, 2000.
T. Wayne Shelton, ed.	*The Ethics of Organ Donation.* New York: Elsevier Science, 2001.
Lee M. Silver	*Remaking Eden: Cloning and Beyond in a Brave New World.* New York: Avon Books, 1997.
Gregory Stock and John Campbell, eds.	*Engineering the Human Germline: An Exploration of the Science and Ethics of Altering the Genes We Pass to Our Children.* New York: Oxford University Press, 2000.
Alan O. Trounson and David K. Gardner, eds.	*Handbook of In Vitro Fertilization.* Boca Raton, FL: CRC Press, 2000.
Stuart J. Youngner, Robert M. Arnold, and Renie Schapiro, eds.	*Definition of Death: Contemporary Controversies.* Baltimore, MD: Johns Hopkins University Press, 1999.

Index